Praise for *Implementing Evidence-Based Practice: Real-Life Success Stories*

"This is a wonderfully engaging and motivational text. I was both monumentally moved and genuinely impressed by these real-life, awe-inspiring stories and the manner in which they so vividly illustrate the human and professional benefits of evidence-based practice. Sincere thanks to all those who so kindly shared their stories, which demonstrate the courage, conviction, and resilience needed to drive EBP steadfastly forward. To Bern and Ellen, thank you for this beautiful string of pearls that no conscientious health care practitioner can afford to be without!"

–Joanne Cleary-Holdforth, RGN, RM, Cert in Renal Nursing,
BSc (Hons), MSc (Hons), PG Dip in Third Level Learning &
Teaching. Cert in EBP Mentorship (ASU)
Lecturer in Nursing, Dublin City University, Ireland

"All too often, the word 'research' causes a nurse's eyes to glaze over. On the other hand, nurses love stories, both to tell and hear. In this book, Melnyk and Fineout-Overholt have very cleverly combined storytelling with research to demonstrate the importance of using evidence to guide nursing care interventions and decision-making. The stories in this collection are by turns compelling, emotional, humorous, and sobering, but all keep evidence-based practice as the primary focus, reinforcing its role as the driver of predictable patient outcomes through high quality care."

–Leslie H. Nicoll, PhD, MBA, RN
Principal and Owner, Maine Desk LLC,
Professional Editorial Services

"This compilation of stories will make a difference in your nursing practice, whether you are a new or seasoned practitioner. These stories provide inspiration and insight into the application of evidence-based practice in the 21st century and make evidence-based practice real for the reader."

–Rita Marie John, DNP, EdD, CPNP
Associate Professor of Clinical Nursing
Columbia University, New York

"If you are looking for a compelling reminder of why evidence-based health care matters for nursing and our patients, read this book. The authors have captured many inspirational stories to lift our spirits and reinvigorate our passion for building our science upon the art of nursing through evidence-based practice. These heartwarming stories are a reminder of the power of nursing."

–Laura Cullen, MA, RN, FAAN
Evidence-Based Practice Coordinator
University of Iowa Hospitals and Clinics

"Drs. Melnyk and Fineout-Overholt have compiled an impressive collection of stories of how nurses use evidence to make a difference and influence care on the front lines. Nurses at all levels of practice will benefit from reading the real-life examples of how their nursing colleagues are putting evidence into practice. This powerful book demonstrates the passion, commitment, and accountability of nurses to patients and to the profession. It delivers a clear message that nurses have a central role in improving health care outcomes by practicing within the framework of evidence-based care."

–Teri Wurmser, PhD, MPH, RN, NEA-BC
Director, Ann May Center for Nursing
Meridian Health, New Jersey

Implementing Evidence-Based Practice

Real-Life Success Stories

Bernadette Mazurek Melnyk, PhD, RN, CPNP/PMHNP, FNAP, FAAN
Ellen Fineout-Overholt, PhD, RN, FNAP, FAAN

Sigma Theta Tau International
Honor Society of Nursing®

The Honor Society of Nursing, Sigma Theta Tau International (STTI) is a nonprofit organization whose mission is to support the learning, knowledge, and professional development of nurses committed to making a difference in health worldwide. Founded in 1922, STTI has 130,000 members in 86 countries. Members include practicing nurses, instructors, researchers, policymakers, entrepreneurs and others. STTI's 470 chapters are located at 586 institutions of higher education throughout Australia, Botswana, Brazil, Canada, Colombia, Ghana, Hong Kong, Japan, Kenya, Malawi, Mexico, The Netherlands, Pakistan, Singapore, South Africa, South Korea, Swaziland, Sweden, Taiwan, Tanzania, the United States and Wales. More information about STTI can be found online at www.nursingsociety.org.

Sigma Theta Tau International
550 West North Street
Indianapolis, IN 46202

To order additional books, buy in bulk, or order for corporate use, contact Nursing Knowledge International at 888.NKI.4YOU (888.654.4968/US and Canada) or +1.317.634.8171 (outside US and Canada).

To request a review copy for course adoption, e-mail solutions@nursingknowledge.org or call 888.NKI.4YOU (888.654.4968/US and Canada) or +1.317.917.4983 (outside US and Canada).

To request author information, or for speaker or other media requests, contact Rachael McLaughlin of the Honor Society of Nursing, Sigma Theta Tau International at 888.634.7575 (US and Canada) or +1.317.634.8171 (outside US and Canada).

ISBN-13:	9781-935476-689
EPUB and Mobi ISBN:	9781-935476-696
PDF ISBN:	9781-935476-702

Library of Congress Cataloging-in-Publication Data

Available via http://catalog.loc.gov/

First Printing, 2011

Publisher: *Renee Wilmeth*
Acquisitions Editors: *Janet Boivin, BSN, RN*
Editorial Coordinator: *Paula Jeffers*
Cover Designer: *Katy Bodenmiller*
Interior Design and Page Composition: *Rebecca Batchelor*

Principal Book Editor: *Carla Hall*
Copy Editor: *Kevin Kent*
Proofreader: *Barbara Bennett*
Indexer: *Johnna Van Hoose Dinse*

Dedication

Bernadette Mazurek Melnyk

I dedicate this book to the awesome nurses and other clinicians who, on a daily basis, dedicate their lives to transforming health and transforming lives by improving the quality of health care and the outcomes of their patients through evidence-based practice (EBP). A chief nursing officer recently told me that the majority of her clinicians were burnt-out and practicing in a coma of complacency, which not only adversely affects their colleagues, but has a detrimental effect on patients. I have seen firsthand throughout the United States and the globe how EBP reignites passion in clinicians and motivates them to deliver a higher quality of care to their patients. I have also seen firsthand how the lack of evidence-based care results in major medical errors, including nearly losing my youngest daughter, which you will read about in the story, entitled "Kaylin's Story: Australian Dream Trip Turned Nightmare." As you read the powerful stories in this book about how clinicians transformed practice and improved their patients' outcomes through EBP, you will reignite your passion for why you first chose your profession and rekindle your commitment to deliver the highest quality of care possible for the benefit of your patients and family members.

Ellen Fineout-Overholt

As I read the stories in this book about how clinicians are making a daily difference in patients', families', and providers' lives, they reinforce my core belief and value of how important each of us is to health care outcomes. My husband and I have two young daughters. I want my children to have health care professionals who care enough about their best outcomes to be the best at what they do (i.e., bring in their expertise); seek out the best science and other knowledge to apply to care; include our daughters' (and our) preferences when making decisions about care; and evaluate whether the treatments, programs, and initiatives they engage actually achieve the expected outcome—that is, I want our daughters to have evidence-based care. This book is dedicated to the nurses who shared their stories with Bern and me and to my precious girls, Rachael and Ruth. I wish you all a long, healthy, vibrant life!

Acknowledgements

Bernadette Mazurek Melnyk

I want to thank and recognize all of the clinicians who contributed their wonderful stories to this book, which I believe is such a treasure. I have been so blessed to travel throughout the United States and the globe, working with nurses and transdisciplinary clinicians in health care systems to advance and sustain evidence-based practice (EBP). What I have learned from them and their stories continually reignites my passion for always working to take our professions to greater heights for the ultimate purpose of enhancing the quality of health care and improving patients' health and lives. I could not accomplish all that I do without the loving support of my husband, John, and my three wonderful daughters, Kaylin, Angela and Megan. They have sacrificed much so that others could benefit, and for that, I can never thank them enough. I also want to thank my very dear friend and colleague, Ellen Fineout-Overholt, for her unwavering commitment over the past 12 years in working tirelessly with me to advance our efforts in improving health care and impacting lives in such a positive way through EBP. I am truly blessed with my family, friendships, and colleagues. In addition, I want to thank and recognize Kathy York, who has been instrumental in the support of my work and a never-failing source of encouragement. Lastly, thanks to the publishing team at Sigma Theta Tau International, including Janet Boivin, Carla Hall, and Renee Wilmeth, who have all been terrific in the production of this work.

Ellen Fineout-Overholt

It was a joy to edit and contribute to this book. It was wonderful to read about evidence-based clinicians making a remarkable difference in how patients and families experience health care and the associated outcomes on a daily basis. I thank each of you for investing in your careers and sharing your stories with others—to inspire, encourage, and challenge us all to provide the best care possible. Special thanks to Kathy York and Debbie Relph for their assistance with e-mails and record keeping. Bern and I are indebted to the publishing team at Sigma Theta Tau International who care so deeply for the nursing profession, particularly Janet Boivin, Carla Hall, and Renee Wilmeth.

Faith, family, and friends —these are why I do what I do. Thank you to those who have prayed for me and this work. Please keep on praying! I so appreciate my wonderful husband and precious girls and their gracious gift of time and sacrifice so that I could work on this book. Finally, Bern, thank you just doesn't cut it. Your vision is extraordinary. Keep dreaming!

About the Authors

Bernadette Mazurek Melnyk, PhD, RN, CPNP/PMHNP, FNAP, FAAN

Bernadette Mazurek Melnyk is currently Dean and Distinguished Foundation Professor at the Arizona State University College of Nursing and Health Innovation. She will assume the position of Associate Vice President for Health Promotion, Chief Wellness Officer, and Dean of the College of Nursing at The Ohio State University in September 2011. She earned her Bachelor of Science in Nursing degree from West Virginia University, her Master of Science in Nursing degree with a specialization in nursing care of children and pediatric nurse practitioner from the University of Pittsburgh, and her PhD in clinical research from the University of Rochester where she also completed her post-master's certificate as a psychiatric mental health nurse practitioner. Dr. Melnyk is a nationally/internationally recognized expert in evidence-based practice, intervention research, and child and adolescent mental health. Her record includes over $11 million of sponsored funding from federal agencies as principal investigator and over 170 publications.

Dr. Melnyk is coeditor of the well-known book, *Evidence-based Practice in Nursing & Healthcare: A Guide to Best Practice* and the *KySS Guide to Child and Adolescent Mental Health Screening, Early Intervention and Health Promotion*. She is a frequent keynote speaker at national and international conferences and has consulted with health care systems and colleges throughout the nation and globe on how to implement and sustain evidence-based practice. Dr. Melnyk is an elected fellow of the American Academy of Nursing and the National Academies of Practice and currently serves as one of only two nurse practitioners on the United States Preventive Services Task Force. She also serves as associate editor of the journal *Worldviews on Evidence-Based Nursing* and is founder of the National Association of Pediatric Nurse Practitioners' KySS Program, a national initiative to promote the mental health of children and teens. Dr. Melnyk has received numerous national and international awards, including the Audrey Hepburn Award from Sigma Theta Tau International; the Jessie Scott Award from the American Nurses Association for the improvement of health care quality through the integration of research, education, and practice; and Sigma Theta Tau International's Research Hall of Fame. She also has been recognized twice as an Edge Runner by the American Academy of Nursing for the KySS Program and her COPE (Creating Opportunities for Parent

Empowerment) Program for parents of premature infants, which has been adopted by insurers and hospitals throughout the nation and globe. In addition, Dr. Melnyk is president of COPE for HOPE, Inc. and partner in ARCC LLC. More information about COPE can be accessed at www.copeforhope.com.

Ellen Fineout-Overholt, PhD, RN, FNAP, FAAN

Dr. Fineout-Overholt is currently Clinical Professor and Director of the Center for the Advancement of Evidence-Based Practice at Arizona State University. Dr. Fineout-Overholt earned her BSN from the University of Texas Medical Branch at Galveston, her MSN in Cardiovascular Nursing from the University of Alabama at Birmingham, and her PhD in Nursing Research from the University of Rochester. Her primary role is assisting health care providers (i.e., nurses, doctors, and other providers) to care for patients using the evidence-based practice (EBP) paradigm, which blends the best scientific information available (i.e., research), the experience of the provider along with evidence from practice, and what patients value and prefer to accomplish the best health outcomes for that patient.

Dr. Fineout-Overholt is best known for promoting EBP with clinicians across the United States and worldwide, both in the hospital and in the community. Dr. Fineout-Overholt, with her long-time colleague Dr. Bernadette Melnyk, developed the **A**dvancing **R**esearch & **C**linical Practice through close **C**ollaboration (**ARCC**) model. This model hinges on the strategic, central role of an EBP mentor to sustain improved health care outcomes. EBP mentors foster an environment that welcomes (a) inquiry; (b) innovation; and (c) solutions that are based on sound scientific and practice-based evidence and focused on improving health care outcomes. EBP mentors, educated in programs created by Dr. Fineout-Overholt, are making a difference in patient and systems outcomes all over the world. In addition, Dr. Fineout-Overholt's innovative work to revise the foundation upon which nurses are educated to integrate EBP principles has been well received by faculty worldwide.

Her publications and presentations, in the United States and abroad, focus on helping clinicians, health care faculty, and administrators improve practice through implementation and sustainability of EBP. Dr. Fineout-Overholt's research is devoted to developing and testing models of EBP in multiple settings. She is coeditor of the widely used book *Evidence-Based Practice in Nursing & Healthcare: A Guide to Best Practice* (Lippincott

Williams & Wilkins), which is in its 2nd edition. Dr. Fineout-Overholt is an elected Fellow in the National Academies of Practice and the American Academy of Nursing and a partner in ARCC LLC. She has received further recognition of her contributions to nursing and the health professions through such honors as the UTMB School of Nursing Distinguished Alumnus for 2009, induction into the UTMB Alumni Association Hall of Fame in 2008, and one of the 60 Visionary Leaders named at the 60th anniversary of University of Alabama Birmingham's School of Nursing in 2010.

Table of Contents

3   Incorporating Patient Preferences and Clinician Expertise in Evidence-Based Practice. 103

Foreword

Across the globe, nurses are striving to improve patients' care and experience through the implementation of evidence-based practice (EBP). As nurses, we all want to do what is right for patients and improve the quality of the care that we deliver. Few would dispute the merit of EBP; it is hard to disagree that we should be providing care based on the best evidence available to us to optimise patient outcomes and maximise health care resources. However, the quest to use evidence and implement best practices often results in complex challenges that have no easy solutions. The publication of this book is therefore timely. What we read on its pages are vivid and realistic stories of nurses' journeys in the implementation of EBP, including both challenges and successes.

Sigma Theta Tau International's 2008 position statement on EBP builds on a previous definition that describes EBP as "a process of shared decision making between practitioner, patient, and others significant to them based on research evidence, the patient's experiences and preferences, clinical expertise or know-how, and other available robust sources of information" (Rycroft-Malone et al., 2004). The outcome of this process could reflect changes in behaviour at individual, team and organisational levels; improvement in individual health outcomes; and better use of resources. What we need to remember, and why the stories of nurses in this book are so important, is that the implementation of EBP is complex, multifaceted, and multilayered. Therefore, any attempt to set out on a journey toward EBP will have numerous obstacles to navigate, bumpy roads to tread, and destinations that are often difficult to foresee.

When reading these chapters one can hear the nurses' voices. These stories cross many clinical topics, contexts, and issues. They represent the gamut of nurses' work life including, for example, peri-operative care, diabetes, breast-feeding, dementia care, COPD, eating disorders, stroke, pain assessment, and cancer care. Metaphors are used to describe the nurses' experiences—particularly the idea of nature and gardens as a way of expressing the fertile ground and flourishing that implementation of evidence-based practices both relies on, and results in. We can see from these examples that delivering EBP can transform nurses, as well as patients.

Common themes emerge from reading these narratives that will be of interest and relevance to others embarking on a similar journey. Unsurprisingly, they also reflect the evidence base about implementation. Research shows us that we need to pay attention to the role that various sources of evidence (internal and external) play in patient-centered decision making, the critical influence that the context of care can play in this process, and the way implementation is planned and facilitated.

Perhaps the starting point, and what we read about in many of these stories, is nurses' spirit of enquiry and ability to reflect on current practice, their passion, and their belief that patient care could be better. If things could be better, then appropriate action is required. This, coupled with genuine stakeholder engagement that includes patients, family members, other nurses, and clinical colleagues, emphasises that what is required for successful implementation is effective teamwork. Furthermore, implementation relies on a clear and planned process that is underpinned by relevant theory and frameworks. But, it also requires a flair for innovation, creative thinking, and flexibility—and the need to slay some sacred cows!

One of the striking issues emerging from these pages is that through the transformation of patient care based on best evidence, nurses also transform their role and experience personal growth. Nurses in these chapters who take leadership and mentorship roles are empowered by their successes and are growing and developing. For me, this demonstrates the transformative effect that EBP implementation can have on nurses as it becomes their "way of life."

Essentially, these accounts celebrate the successes of nurses. Their stories serve to inspire, encourage, and empower us all to realise that as nurses, we can make a difference in patient care—which, after all, is the ultimate goal of implementing EBP.

–Jo Rycroft-Malone, PhD, MSc, BSc (Hons), RN
Professor, Bangor University, United Kingdom
Editor, Worldviews on Evidence-Based Nursing

References

Rycroft-Malone, J., Seers, K., Titchen, A., Harvey, G., Kitson, A., & McCormack, B. (2004). What counts as evidence in evidence-based practice? Journal of Advanced Nursing, 47(1), 81-90.

Sigma Theta Tau International 2005-2007. (2008). Research and scholarship advisory committee position statement 2008. Worldviews on Evidence-Based Nursing, 5(2), 57-59.

Introduction

Although studies have supported that evidence-based practice (EBP) enhances health care quality, reduces costs, and improves patient outcomes, the majority of clinicians are not consistently implementing EBP. Further, many health care systems across the nation and globe do not have cultures to support the sustainability of EBP by clinicians. Unfortunately, there remains a large time gap between the translation of research findings into clinical practice to improve care and outcomes. Therefore, to reach the Institute of Medicine's goal that by 2020, 90% of health care decisions be evidence-based, intense efforts to enhance and sustain EBP must be implemented in health care systems across the United States.

Evidence-based practice is a problem-solving approach to the delivery of care that integrates the best evidence from a body of studies with a clinician's expertise, which includes internal evidence and patient assessments, and a patient's preferences and values. The goal of this lifelong learning approach is the achievement of outcomes that are right for a particular patient. The decision-making happens within a context of caring, enabling each provider-patient encounter to be as unique as it is and deliver unique outcomes (see Figure 1).

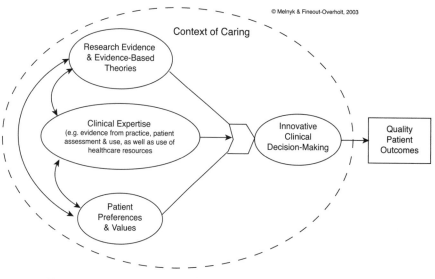

Figure 1.1   EBP Paradigm Conceptual Framework

The EBP process contains seven steps that range from igniting inquiry to sharing results of practice changes, large and small, with others who can benefit from them (see upcoming sidebar). This process is meant to be engaged within the EBP paradigm (i.e., the way we think about our practice). For the EBP process to fully impact practice, this conceptual framework must be in place; that is, clinicians must include research, their expertise, and the patients values and preferences in their daily clinical decision making for the purpose of achieving the agreed upon outcome; otherwise, the EBP process becomes just a process and is not sustainable .

The Seven Steps of the EBP Process

Step 0: Cultivate a spirit of inquiry

Step 1: Ask the clinical question in PICOT (Patient population; Intervention or area of Interest; Comparison intervention or group; Outcome; Time) format

Step 2: Search for and collect the most relevant and best evidence to answer the clinical question

Step 3: Critically appraise the evidence: First rapidly appraise the evidence that has been collected for its validity, reliability, and applicability; then evaluate it for how it best answers the question; then synthesize that evidence to determine what is known from that body of evidence

Step 4: Integrate the evidence with one's clinical expertise and the patient's preferences and values to implement a clinical decision

Step 5. Evaluate outcomes of the practice decision or change based on evidence

Step 6. Disseminate the outcomes of the EBP decision or change

© Melnyk & Fineout-Overholt 2011

Although multiple barriers exist to the consistent implementation of EBP in health care systems, facilitators can help to advance and sustain EBP, which include (a) strong beliefs by clinicians that EBP improves care and patient outcomes; (b) knowledge and skills in EBP; (c) EBP mentors (i.e., typically clinicians with strong knowledge and skills in EBP, along with skills in individual and organizational behavior change); (d) EBP resources and tools; and (e) administrators who support EBP and who model it. It must be remembered that information alone does not typically change behavior. Most people, including clinicians, do not change behavior until a crisis happens or they experience an emotional impact that gets their attention. One of the key purposes of this book is to connect with clinicians' emotions as they read these stories so that they are compelled to learn more about EBP and to initiate evidence-based care because it leads to better outcomes for their patients and families.

The inspiration for this book is our love of stories and how the telling of them can make such a difference in how people connect with the concepts of evidence-based practice (EBP). We use stories all of the time in our work. Stories help us see concepts in a new light. If we see concepts operationalized in stories, we have more confidence that we can make them work for us.

To make this book a reality, we disseminated a national call for EBP stories that would touch the heart or appeal to the emotions of health care providers. Our desire was for clinicians to share their experiences with paradigm shifts to EBP, implementation of the EBP process to change practice and improve patient outcomes, personal experiences with evidence-based care, and transforming systems to an EBP culture. The result is 90 stories from 27 states across the nation and one story from Canada that reflect a commitment to quality, safe, and cost-efficient care through EBP.

Because these are stories and we are committed to preserving the authors' voices, the editing was minimal and solely for the purpose of enhancing clarity of the story. Because these are stories, there are no references in this book. If you read a story that particularly inspires you, we encourage you to contact the authors. Our dream is that clinicians will keep sharing their stories and further change will occur.

The book is organized around the EBP paradigm and the seven steps of the EBP process. Both begin with a spirit of inquiry. There are 20 stories in Chapter 1 that inspire and demonstrate how to foster a spirit of inquiry in health care. Chapter 2 is dedicated to innovation in health care, with 15 studies shedding light on how clinicians can improve care with unique evidence-based ideas. Chapter 3 includes 9 stories about the critical importance of combining patient preferences and values with the expertise of the clinician and external evidence as clinical decisions are made. Chapter 4 reflects the impact of EBP on outcomes through 27 wonderful stories. Given that outcomes are the "bottom line" of health care, this chapter is particularly important to the core of the mission of the book—to help you, the reader, experience the reality of the impact of EBP. Chapter 5 offers 9 stories about how team work accomplishes more when implementing evidence-based change. Finally, Chapter 6 contains 9 stories that provide insight into how to mentor and teach others about EBP, which is foundational to a successful EBP culture.

The stories in this book were written by real people, just like you, who have made a positive difference in their patients' lives. Sometimes making the difference was the job for the day. In other cases, the difference was serendipitous. Whatever your role in health care, as you read these stories, we hope that they inspire you and that you are encouraged to dream, innovate, and persist in making a positive impact, a difference—today, tomorrow, and beyond. We suggest that you first read the stories through, chapter by chapter. As you read, select your favorites that particularly inspire you. Mark them so that you can return to them again and again. Give the book to others who you know will be inspired by the stories. As you read these stories, you may be spurred on to write your own story; please do so and send it along to us as we compile Volume II of *Implementing Evidence-based Practice: Real-Life Success Stories*. We hope that as you read the stories you will realize that we are all on the same journey and that each of us is contributing to the mission of evidence-based patient care that reaps the best outcomes for our patients and families.

Bern & Ellen
Bern@transforminghealthcarewitharcc.com
Ellen@transforminghealthcarewitharcc.com

Igniting Passion and a Spirit of Inquiry With Evidence-Based Practice

Anything is possible with a big dream, passion, and the courage to persist through the character-building events that will undoubtedly occur in your pursuit of the dream. Passion is necessary to succeed at any endeavor, including the delivery of high quality care through evidence-based practice (EBP).

The very first step in EBP (Step 0) is igniting a spirit of inquiry, a never-ending curiosity about the care that is being delivered and its associated outcomes. When clinicians have a spirit of inquiry, they are constantly asking questions about the care they are providing to their patients, the outcomes it achieves, and the evidence to support that care (e.g., in children with asthma, how does the use of a metered-dose inhaler with spacer versus a nebulizer to deliver a bronchidilater affect oxygen saturation and time in the emergency room?). This spirit of inquiry is necessary to progress to Step #1 of EBP, which is asking questions in PICOT (Patient Population; Intervention or interest area; Comparison intervention or group; Outcome; Time) format.

The stories in this chapter provide wonderful exemplars of how a spirit of inquiry by clinicians ignited improvements in patient care and outcomes through EBP. The passion that these clinicians had for their EBP journeys is evident. The stories also illustrate how EBP can reignite passion and enthusiasm in clinicians who had lost them.

It All Began With a Student Nurse

–Judi Schofield, MSN, RN, NE-BC
Manager, Cardiovascular Step-down Unit
The Christ Hospital, Cincinnati, Ohio

"Why did you tell that patient to remain in bed for 2 hours?" the student nurse asked her preceptor one Monday afternoon as they were walking down the hallway. They had just removed the temporary epicardial pacing wires from an open-heart surgery patient who was preparing for discharge the following day and were discussing the process with each other. This was the beginning of the biggest practice change on our unit that improved quality of care for patients and laid the foundation for a culture of evidence-based practice (EBP) for the nurses.

"Because that's the way I was taught," the nurse replied nonchalantly. The student pressed on. "But why 2 hours?" she persisted. The staff nurse realized she didn't have a valid answer, so she began to survey the rest of the staff. The responses were surprising as the resting time reported by the nurses varied from 15 minutes to 3 hours, but the basis of all the answers was always the same: "Because that is what my preceptor told me."

Our 550-bed community hospital was known for its outstanding cardiac care, so the staff took their role in quality of care seriously. We realized that we had no consistent activity protocol post-pacing-wire removal, and we were engaging in a practice that had no scientific origin but was based in a unit tradition passed down over time. We even asked the cardiac surgeons for their opinion, and they thought that maybe the practice originated from a case back in 1986 when a patient had developed cardiac tamponade after removal of the wires. It was determined that bedrest might prevent this from happening again, but no one could validate that fact or the difference in rest times.

The controversy stirred some interesting conversation, so we decided to do a literature search to see what other nurses were doing. We discovered that there wasn't much written on the topic, and what was available was geared toward physicians and not nurses. "Let's do our own study," I said enthusiastically. I was the manager of this cardiovascular step-down unit, and though I didn't know much about EBP, the organization had recently asked us to begin to incorporate it into our protocols. I saw this as an opportunity to begin that process.

It took some initial convincing, but eventually the staff got excited because they saw that they could do something that influenced their practice. With the blessing of the Institutional Review Board and the surgeons, we conducted a small, unit-based study that compared the effect of activity after pacing-wire removal to bedrest. We drew a number for each patient before each procedure, and the even-numbered patients were told to remain in bed for 30 minutes, while the odd-numbered ones were ambulated around the unit after the removal. A total of 60 patients participated in the study, and the results showed no difference in the outcomes of either group. Since Coumadin was an exclusion criterion in the initial study, we conducted a second one with patients on that drug. The outcome was the same; no difference. We took the results to the unit-based council, and a new evidence-based protocol that included no activity restrictions after the removal of temporary pacing wires was put into place.

Despite the results, it was unclear if the practice actually changed or if attitudes about EBP increased. Currently, it often takes more than a decade to move nursing research to the bedside, so we wondered if being involved in a unit-based study made the results more relevant to the nurses. A follow-up anonymous questionnaire was collected to get feedback from the staff nurses involved. Ninety-three percent of the staff nurses said that being involved in this process made the results more relevant and that they integrated the changes into their practice. Some of the comments written on the questionnaire demonstrate the effectiveness of this project:

> "I found the study to be a great hands-on way to learning about how to do research and how the findings can be put into practice."

> "Not only did this study provide a scientific-based foundation for pulling pacing wires, but it provides our patients safe care."

> "I was happy to be involved in the research study. I like being able to improve patient outcomes."

The drive to take nursing from a traditional base to one of evidence is increasing. Making the change from the academic level to the clinical side has been slow and tedious. In order to move evidence-based findings into practice, it is essential to begin at the bedside. Involving staff nurses in studies that affect their daily practice was a successful paradigm shift on this unit, and it all began with a question from a student nurse.

Each unit in each institution conducting bedside studies will only spark more studies, and the results can be shared among all nurses. Now on this cardiovascular step-down unit, every time a question is raised about a practice process, the response is, "Let's find the evidence!"

Although this was a small, unit-based study, it is significant to nursing practice. It is the catalyst for nursing to understand that if it wants to change to a profession based in evidence, it must first begin with the stakeholders who are invested in the outcome: the staff nurses.

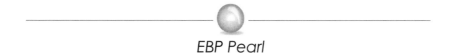

EBP Pearl

Involvement of bedside staff as stakeholders in EBP and research projects will ignite a spirit of inquiry and speed the acceleration of evidence-based practice to improve patient outcomes.

Evidence-Based Practice . . . A Spirit of Inquiry

–Karen Sakakeeny, BSN, RN, CNOR, CPN
Staff Nurse Level III, Main Operating Room
Children's Hospital Boston, Boston, Massachusetts

Looking back on my 32 years of nursing practice at Children's Hospital Boston, I realize now that evidence-based practice (EBP) has always been diffused throughout my clinical career. I have always been self-motivated and actively open to learning new skills. During my evolution from novice to expert, I can proudly say that I initiated and assumed a leadership role in the research and development of several standards of patient care while embracing our Synergy model. I always managed to seek out the sickest patient population and more complex procedures that were extremely challenging. I have been instrumental in orchestrating and developing our solid organ transplant program, extracorporeal membrane oxygenation (ECMO), and fetal surgery program while working in the operating room (OR) for the last 30 years. Moreover, I was the first RN who independently pursued peripherally inserted central line (PICC line) certification in the perioperative arena, enabling patients to receive PICC lines while under general anesthesia. My most recent achievement, publishing in the *American Journal of Nursing*, is truly the pinnacle in demonstrating my determination to accomplish a professional dream. However, articulating and implementing the EBP process at the point of care was what my practice lacked.

My EBP journey began in 2006, before I even understood its concepts and framework. It was set in motion one day when I was precepting a colleague in the main OR (MOR). Although most of our pediatric patients in the MOR have procedures requiring general anesthesia, occasionally some patients receive local anesthesia. When this occurs, there is no anesthesiologist attending to the patient, only one nurse in the circulating role, and the other nurse is scrubbed at the sterile field with the surgeons. My last two cases of the day were scheduled for biopsies under local anesthesia; because there were two of us (my orientee and me), I decided to delegate the role of circulating nurse to my orientee. My sole mission would be to stay completely with the conscious patient from beginning to end, monitoring and comforting. While sitting with each patient at the head of the bed, I became acutely aware how busy the circulating nurse was during each case. Because my orientee was there to help, I could focus my attention on assessing and monitoring the patient's physiologic and psychological needs while my orientee tended to the other responsibilities pertaining to the circulating role. At the end of both local procedures, the surgeon commented on how well both cases went and said that he could not have done it without me continuously by each patient's side distracting, supporting, encouraging, and bonding with them. The positive outcome for the patient and the staff satisfaction was remarkable.

As I reflected on this experience, I was convinced that having two RNs circulating for patients receiving local anesthesia should be our standard of care. I wanted to change our practice to make it mandatory for a second circulating RN to be assigned for supporting and monitoring the patient receiving local anesthesia. My intuitive clinical expertise to do the right thing at the right time for the right patient population was valid.

However, I lacked knowledge of a model to help support and integrate this practice change with the best external clinical evidence.

A week later, I attended a perioperative retreat where one of the main topics was EBP. As I listened to the presenters and learned more about EBP, I realized how my experience with patients receiving local anesthesia was a perfect venue to make a practice change using EBP. I recognized how the EBP process is a practical approach to implement change in clinical practice while demonstrating accountability. I regularly exhibited clinical inquiry by questioning and evaluating our current practice, but lacked a tool that would help me structure how to make decisions in my clinical practice that were correct and how to apply evidence in the practice setting. I found it within the EBP domain. Learning that EBP is the conscientious use of current best evidence in making decisions about patient care allowed me to legitimately pursue my goal of having two RNs circulating for patients receiving local anesthesia as our standard of care.

Following the retreat, I joined the Perioperative EBP Committee, where I received wonderful leadership support from my colleagues who helped me with the evidence review and expertly guided me in the process of implementing informed practice. I then wrote a revised policy for patients undergoing procedures with local anesthesia that was supported by the evidence I had appraised and referenced.

I presented my new policy to the Perioperative Practice Committee. They supported this change 100%. It was approved by our director of Perioperative Programs and Allied Services and was added to our Net Learning requirements so staff would be educated about the new policy for *Recommended Practices for Managing the Patient Receiving Local Anesthesia*. The feedback after implementation was extremely positive. Surgeons expressed their satisfaction with the process and remarked that they could not have done the procedure as quickly and as smoothly with only one nurse assigned to the patient. In the past, they had to stop often to console, assure, and instruct the patient. Furthermore, the surgeons noted that their concentration was better because the patient was less upset during the procedure. Another benefit to the circulating nurses was they could fulfill their role on the surgical team, focusing on obtaining needed supplies, providing assistance, and maintaining overall management of the room, rather than consoling the patient. The perioperative RN is ultimately accountable for the patient outcomes resulting from the nursing care provided during the surgical or invasive procedure. The

Association of PeriOperative Nurses (AORN) states that the goal of perioperative nursing practice is to assist patients and their families to achieve a level of wellness equal to or greater than that which they had before the procedure. Nursing colleagues mentioned they were less stressed because they could better accomplish this practice goal. In addition, several parents commented their child actually had "fun" in the OR!

AORN holds a strong position on dedicating one perioperative registered circulating nurse to every patient undergoing a surgical or other invasive procedure. This practice change enabled us to better follow this guideline and deliver care in accordance with the principles of child development. Consequently, the main outcomes of this project are improved satisfaction for patients receiving local anesthesia and improved perioperative staff satisfaction.

In October of 2009, I was selected by my nurse manager to participate in The Peri-Operative Evidence-Based Practice Internship. This internship was a pilot study developed and spearheaded by Linda Connor, MHA, RN, CPN, and Natalie McClain, PhD, RN, with the goal of all participants becoming mentors in our individual areas to promote EBP in nursing practice. I believe my previous experience with EBP helped qualify me to meet the expectations of this course and be chosen as one of the participants. I partnered with a colleague and began my vigorous and challenging journey into learning and understanding the "real deal" of EBP. By the end of the course, we were successful in accessing the EBP support services at Children's Hospital Boston. We then developed and answered a clinical question based on best evidence and completed an EBP project. Upon completion, we developed a PowerPoint presentation and disseminated our information to our department. Ultimately, we went on to create and present a poster of our project for Nurses Week in May 2010. The energy that came out of this project propelled us further. We are now in the beginning stages of initiating and potentially developing a small pilot research study for improved patient outcomes and our own experience as health care consumers.

What has helped me the most in this journey is realizing that EBP is *not* research. We might find opportunities to conduct research after our EBP project, but an EBP project is to look at what evidence is already out there and figure out how to translate that into practice. Understanding this concept completely changed my outlook and focus on incorporating EBP into my clinical nursing practice. It inspired me to realize from my heart that EBP is an intricate part of my job as a practicing nurse at Children's Hospital

Boston. Moreover, EBP has encouraged me to develop a more innovative practice and capture a spirit of independence and determination, allowing me to voluntarily strive to fulfill goals and initiate necessary practice changes.

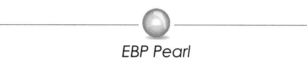

EBP Pearl

Learn, grow, observe, act, evaluate . . . Just do EBP!

Who Would Have Known . . .

–Monica T. Majercin, BSN, RN
Intensive Care Unit
Banner Baywood Medical Center, Mesa, Arizona

When my youngest child was diagnosed with Type 1 diabetes at the age of 5, my interest in insulin and blood sugar control peaked, needless to say! We poked her little fingers 6–8 times a day, injected her with insulin 4–5 times a day, and maintained her happy-go-lucky spirit. As a nurse and a mother, I thought there must be a better/easier way to manage a child's blood sugar and insulin delivery. I was aware of the insulin pump and the evidence that utilizing the pump had a positive outcome in glucose control. Unfortunately, I was told that the pump was not being used in prepubescent adolescents because of the hormonal and blood sugar changes that occur with puberty.

Fortunately, we were partnered with a champion pediatric endocrinologist who was willing to study this population and the outcomes of the insulin pump. My daughter participated in the study when she was 12 years old. The evidence demonstrated that utilizing the insulin pump afforded better blood sugar control and decreased the glycosolated hemoglobin. My daughter is now 21 years old and has been "pumping" ever since that study. Little did I know almost 10 years ago that I was actively involved in and passionate about what is now called evidence-based practice! But it works and is still working on a very personal level in our home.

Now, many years later, I am still passionate about blood sugars and intensive insulin therapy and am learning more about using EBP in my nursing care. My influence is helping others, too, as two of my colleagues and I presented *Managing Serum Glucose Levels in Critically Ill Adults: Nursing Strategies and Outcome* at one of the evidence-based practice conferences in Phoenix, Arizona.

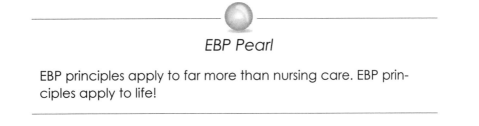

EBP Pearl

EBP principles apply to far more than nursing care. EBP principles apply to life!

A New Way of Life

–Marilyn G. Beller, RN, CAPA, CCRN Alumnus
Staff Nurse III, Ambulatory Surgery,
Department of Perioperative Services
University Medical Center, Tucson, Arizona

The majority of my 48-year career as a nurse was spent in cardiac intensive care. It was in a university medical center with the latest medications, equipment, and techniques being used, trialed, and researched. We were the home of the CardioWest artificial heart and the only transplant center in the state. I had the joy of belonging to the MOBI transport team. We traveled around the state and nearby states rescuing cardiac patients that could benefit from the expertise and cardiac devices that were available only at our center. I learned to value the research-based care we gave, and also the continuing research and trialing that we did at the center. I am still a member of the American Association of Critical-Care Nurses and was a critical care registered nurse for 21 years.

When my body continued to complain about the physical rigors of the high acuity intensive care unit (ICU), I found that I had to make a decision. I was still very much a nurse and wanted to care for patients. I still wanted to come to work to get my "patient fix." I had said for years that when I could no longer practice in the ICU I would like to transfer to ambulatory surgery. No beds to push to CT and MRI. No every 2 hours pulling patients up in bed and turning. No more loading our 350# MOBI into airplanes or ambulances. How sad, as I still loved that kind of practice, but my body didn't love it any more.

When I transferred to ambulatory surgery, I joined the American Society of Peri-Anesthesia Nurses and started working on becoming certified as an Ambulatory PeriAnesthesia Nurse (CAPA). I also continued participation in all of my hospital-wide committees. It was at our Standards of Care Committee that I first learned to conduct evidence-based searches. We created evidence-based standards. No more doing it *just because we always did it that way*. After a Joint Commission visit, we had a year or so before we needed to review the standards and update them. Our chairperson challenged us to pick an issue relevant to our area of practice. Then we were instructed to search out the evidence to support or change the issue.

For many years, I wondered why if NPO after Midnight worked for the 7:30 A.M. surgical case it was necessary for the 3:00 P.M. case. In the ambulatory surgery preoperative area, I frequently heard my patients complain of being hungry and thirsty. Certainly, water didn't hang around in your stomach for 8 hours when you obviously were dehydrated. It seemed a little ridiculous for the newbie (me!) in the department to be looking at the long "sacred cow" policy. It was the standard when I graduated from nursing in 1962. Now, it was 2005. So, I set out to find the evidence out there waiting for me to discover it.

I chose NPO after Midnight as my area of inquiry and search topic! I began checking all of my familiar places to find evidence, including the National Guideline Clearinghouse, the New Zealand Guidelines Group, Agency for Healthcare Research & Quality, Google, Ovid, and the Cochrane Database of Systematic Reviews. The first thing that I discovered was no evidence existed out there to answer my question. Absolutely nothing! So, I changed my question from NPO after Midnight to Preoperative Fasting. I started my search again and BINGO! I was able to find Level I evidence, the highest level of evidence to guide clinical practice, that included meta-analyses and evidence-based guidelines along with a properly designed randomized controlled trial, which is Level II evidence. I also found that the American Society of Anesthesiologists (ASA) had written *Practice Guidelines for Preoperative Fasting* in 1999. I started gathering my evidence in 2005.

From the evidence, I learned that you actually have a larger volume of contents after 6 hours of clear liquid fasting than after 2 hours. The evidence also supported that black coffee, tea, or caffeine-rich sodas help patients avoid a caffeine-withdrawal headache. Plus, just being able to eat Jell-O, drink broth, or have a Popsicle did wonders for the patient. It also helped to start IVs when the patient was not so dry. Further, if the clears were carbohydrate rich, they reduced the catabolic response (insulin resistance) postoperatively. Also, the quality of clears (e.g., no cream or milk products) was what mattered, not the quantity. Findings from research also showed that the body can handle quarts as easily as ounces and stated that people are more compliant if they understand the rationale behind why they are asked to do something.

After reviewing the evidence, I decided that I would present the evidence to the chief of anesthesia at my hospital. I honestly doubted the chance of changing our sacred cow practice, but I was going to give it my best shot. Off I went, armed to present my evidence to the Chief's office, including the anesthesia director of the operating room (OR) and the medical director of the OR. It resulted in nothing, absolutely nothing! I am not sure if they even read it. I should have read it to them with all the enthusiasm I had for what I had found. Well, I tried, and I continued to believe we needed to change and to update our practice with the latest evidence.

One of my nursing colleagues was on a task force looking at expediting our OR services. She overheard one of our anesthesiologists expressing an interest in looking at what evidence was available regarding fasting guidelines. She wasted no time in sharing with him that I had gathered the data. She asked if he would be interested in seeing it. Of course, he gave a resounding "Yes!"

Within a few short weeks, we had a new NPO guideline in print for us to use. It took about a year to get the NPO guideline policy rewritten and approved through the channels. That was the easy part. That was when the work of implementing it really began. It has been a slow, gradual learning curve for everyone, including the nurses, anesthesiologists, surgeons, and patients.

Our preoperative clinic had to be convinced that it was a very safe, evidence-based policy. If the staff in the clinic does not follow it, we are not compliant with written hospital policy. It took about a year to become compliant. We began telling patients that they could have breakfast at 6:00 A.M. if they were having surgery at 2:00 P.M., or they could get up at 4:30 A.M. and have black coffee or broth or Jell-O if they are a 7:30 A.M. case. Our clinic now tells patients that they can have clears up until 3 hours before they are scheduled for survey. We allow an extra hour in case we can take them earlier than scheduled.

Our anesthesiologists, especially the old school ones, did not want to hear about the change, let alone read that the ASA had recommended the changes in protocol since 1999. Absolutely no way were they going to give monitored anesthesia care (MAC) or try to intubate a patient that had a glass of water or coffee 2–3 hours ago! Our OR Chief of Anesthesia helped to coauthor the new policy and stood behind it 100%. Thanks to his strong leadership the policy was enacted and enforced. We were instructed to call him if we encountered an anesthesiologist who refused to perform a case. Our chief would become the responsible attending. He had written the policy and believed in it.

We also have conducted teaching with the office staff of the surgeons. However, the surgeons are still learning that we would prefer that their offices do not tell the patient "nothing by mouth" after midnight. Our clinic calls and gives the patients our guidelines. However, many patients still receive conflicting information from the surgeon's office staff. Unfortunately, they usually follow their surgeon's advice, even when we tell them why they can eat and drink. The patient does not typically understand that it is the anesthesiologist who takes care of them while their surgeon is doing his or her thing. We also have worked with the units/floors to help the staff realize what the hospital policy says about fasting prior to surgery. They are getting better about giving the patients their medications prior to surgery, but it is usually with sips of water. However, I console myself with the fact that their oral medications are current, not held since midnight.

When the patients follow our evidence-based guideline, we in the preoperative ready room (holding) get to reap the benefits of happy patients. No caffeine headaches and usually no dehydration issues, including thirst and shrunken veins for IV starts. We have less psychological and physiological issues when the guideline is followed.

All in all, it has been a rewarding experience. That this old school nurse could be actively involved with using evidence to change a policy that positively affects the patient population of our hospital feels like a real accomplishment. I could not have done it without all who gathered and published research, as well as those who believed what

I gathered and used their powers to change practice. Since this experience, I have been involved with rewriting our home care instructions and handouts for our ambulatory surgery department. Guess what? We use evidence to guide our practices whenever we can find it. It is now a way of life.

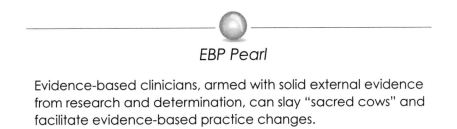

EBP Pearl

Evidence-based clinicians, armed with solid external evidence from research and determination, can slay "sacred cows" and facilitate evidence-based practice changes.

The Itch Factor

–*Jennifer M. Brewer, BSN, RN, CNRN, Research Nurse Coordinator*
–*Paula F. Coe, MSN, RN, NEA-BC, Director of Patient Care Services*
–*Karen Clark, BSN, RN-C, Birthplace Clinical Nurse*
Holy Spirit Hospital, Camp Hill, Pennsylvania
–*Nancy Woods, PhD, MPH, RN, Associate Professor*
Messiah College, Grantham, Pennsylvania

Early in 2009, clinical nurses in the Birthplace (maternity unit) were asking themselves what they could do to improve the pruritis that was plaguing their postpartum, Cesarean section (C-section) mothers. They were noticing that the mothers were having a difficult time with breastfeeding, and newborns were lethargic and not latching on appropriately. The nurses felt this was a side effect of the mothers receiving diphenhydramine (Benadryl) for itching after receiving Duramorph to help control postoperative surgical pain for their C-section. The antihistamines were being passed to the newborns during breastfeeding, leading to their difficulty with latching on as well as irritability with the infants. More importantly, the nurses noticed that Benadryl given to the mothers was not helping to relieve the problem for which it was prescribed because the mothers were still complaining of itching.

The clinical nurses were aware that Benadryl was not working by using their critical-thinking skills and observation of this patient population over several months to years of this practice. They asked themselves what they could do to help advocate for the mothers who were sleepy, tired, stressed, and still itching. The clinical staff questioned how they could impact the outcomes for successful breastfeeding as well as be patient advocates for mothers with significant pruritis. The nurses were searching for a way to deal with this clinical problem. Use of nursing research and an evidence-based practice (EBP) framework and platform was just beginning in the hospital. We had just hired a research nurse coordinator to help facilitate, implement, and coordinate projects by and for the nursing staff. Mary Williams, a Birthplace RN, shared her concerns during an education and research council meeting. The research nurse coordinator and Birthplace nurse made an appointment to discuss and bring to life the EBP project, exploring this clinical question.

Around the same time, we had entered into a relationship with Messiah College, a local school of nursing. During beginning discussions with the nursing department at the college, we identified a nursing research consultant, Nancy Woods, PhD, MPH, RN, who has expertise in the use of the Johns Hopkins EBP Model. With her doctoral work and clinical background in midwifery, Dr. Woods was an enthusiastic, eager partner and collaborator in the first project to help the clinical nurses translate their clinical question into evidence and improve outcomes for this patient population.

The EBP team formed included Mary Williams, RN-C; Karen Clark, BSN, RN-C, from the Birthplace; Jenny Brewer, BSN, RN, CNRN, Research Nurse Coordinator; Paula Coe, MSN, RN, NEA-BC, Director of Nursing; Charlotte Wool, MSN, RN; Dr. Woods; and Edie Asbury, MLS, AHIP, the medical librarian. Edie Asbury assisted with the literature search, and Dr. Woods taught the nurses how to begin to search the literature and available databases for evidence using the tools available in the library. The team utilized the John Hopkins model to critically appraise the literature and decide on the levels of evidence for each article reviewed.

The group met on a monthly basis to develop the project. We began by identifying the problem as Duramorph-induced pruritis in post-C-section mothers. Dr. Woods explained that the Johns Hopkins EBP forms helped to identify a search strategy and critically appraise the literature. Edie Asbury assisted in obtaining appropriate articles for critical appraisal. The list of articles related to Duramorph-induced pruritis was first widened to include all types of epidurals, but later excluded everything but those dealing with C-sections. The sample size also was a determining factor in refining the list. The journals were dated between 1996 and 2008. This time frame was chosen because of the lack of evidence found within the past 5 years. All articles were peer-reviewed, and the bibliographies from the articles were hand searched, which was helpful in finding other relevant literature. We found 20 articles related to the problem and, after review, found eight that addressed our specific problem. These eight articles were critically appraised by the group.

Each team member critically appraised two articles. We identified six Level I articles with an A quality. We had no Level II or Level III articles. We had one Level IV article with an A quality and one Level V article with a C quality. The literature review revealed that Benadryl was completely ineffective in treating the itching from the Duramorph. Although Nalbuphine, Odansetron, and Narcan were identified as treatments for opioid-induced pruritis, findings from the studies indicated that Narcan 0.2–0.25 mcg/kg/hour was the most effective treatment. Narcan in small doses inhibited the mu-opioid receptors successfully, treating the itching without side effects to the newborns as had been seen with the Benadryl. The clinical nurses were thrilled to discover that what they had thought all along had been supported with a search for the evidence. They could now propose a change in practice through translation of this knowledge that could positively impact their patients' outcomes, including reducing itching and improving breastfeeding. An abstract was developed with recommendations for a change in practice.

With their new knowledge and abstract in hand, the clinical nurses set out and made appointments with the unit practice council, anesthesiologists, and OB/GYN physicians to present their findings. They presented their findings at the physician department meetings, proposing the use of Narcan based on evidence from the research literature. The physicians were intrigued with the process the clinical nurses and team had used and were complimentary of their advocacy on behalf of their patients. The physicians agreed to the proposed changes.

Within 6 months of their initial question, the clinical nurses in the Birthplace managed to change practice using evidence-based orders to control pruritis and eliminate the problem new mothers were having with breastfeeding. The nurses changed their documentation flow sheet to assess each mother's pruritis using a Likert scale and are using the information to evaluate the change in practice. They are consulting and utilizing the lactation consultant on a more consistent basis, along with using their assessment skills and nursing interventions to deal with any breastfeeding problems.

The next step will be a research project related to the effects of itching on the post-C-section patient. During the evidence search, it was inferred that itching was not a life or death symptom and, therefore, did not have much significance. The clinical nurses were concerned with this statement, noting that the authors probably had never seen a patient with pruritis to the extreme where it created a physical malady. The clinical nurses were so distressed by this inference that they have begun working on a nursing research proposal to explore the significance of itching in the postpartum C-section patient.

Since this EBP project has been completed, the clinical nurses presented their work at Nursing Grand Rounds as well as at the South Central EBP Consortium, an organization that is a regional collaboration between academic and acute care organizations designed to address and facilitate the promotion of EBP. In this forum, the clinical nurses disseminated the findings to their nursing colleagues, further demonstrating and providing a venue through which their new knowledge could affect patient outcomes in other practice settings. This project has helped to demonstrate how to use the Johns Hopkins EBP Model as a means to critically appraise the literature. We operationalize our shared governance structure by having clinical questions asked in the council forum and using our infrastructure within nursing and research to provide support to answer those questions. We developed a strong collaborative relationship with our research consultant and Messiah College and continue to expand upon this partnership through our Collaborating on Research Evidence (CORE) Essentials program with our clinical nurses and senior year Messiah College nursing students.

EBP Pearl

Partnerships between hospitals/health care systems and academia can accelerate EBP and be a win-win for both institutions and for patients.

Planting Seeds and Watching Our Garden Grow

–Deborah Burgoon, MS, RN, AOCN
–Martha Buffum, DNSc, RN, PMHCNS-BC
–Jane Rudolph, MBA, RN, BA
–Kristi Haney Chambers, MS, RNw, PMHCNS-BC
–Alicia Levin, MS, RN, BA
–Mimi Haberfelde, MS, RN-BC
–Diane Bedecarré, MS, RN-BC
Veterans Affairs Medical Center,
San Francisco, California

Once upon a time, a young nurse said, "I'm bored; I don't feel challenged. I feel like all I do is tasks!" Unfortunately, she left our hospital. We lost an important seedling. Fearful that more seedlings would join her and our garden would not grow, we knew we had to reevaluate nutrients in our soil. And so our EBP story begins.

Deborah, our oncology clinical specialist, had an idea. She read an article about bringing evidence-based practice (EBP) to the unit level. As she works on the oncology-specialized medical-surgical unit, she wanted to replicate methods described in that article to her unit. With her excellent relationships with the unit staff, she was ideally situated to make this a successful project.

At the onset, Deborah gathered her team, first seeking Marti, our associate chief nurse for research. Together, they identified key team players—Alicia, Mimi, Diane, Kristi. We brainstormed, made a plan, laughed a lot, thought about the use of humor and art, and decided what was needed to make the garden grow. Overall, we knew we needed rich soil, good seeds, water and nutrients, and nurturing for a productive garden.

Brainstorming sessions nurtured our soil with good ideas for proceeding. We thought if nurses were provided stimulation and support, they could enrich their practice. Our unit had nurses with varying levels of experience and education, inconsistent practices, insufficient organizational support, inadequate knowledge of available resources, and lack of knowledge about seeking and critically appraising literature. Our beliefs were that nurses would engage in EBP if we acquired organizational support, provided educational fertilizer, and offered resources, assistance, and ongoing sustenance.

We gathered our finest seeds. We started with the unit nurse manager who was supportive and willing to provide staff with participation time. We shared the plan, obtaining support from nursing administration. Alicia, Mimi, and Diane produced creative poster art using a Sherlock Holmes theme to pique curiosity. They created guessing games with treasure hunts and evoked lots of laughter and intrigue while nurses solved the mysteries. We created invitations to a series of classes that would attract the nurse detectives. We were developing seedlings as we enriched the soil with new nutrients.

As of January 2005, we were a team of three clinical nurse specialists (oncology, diabetes, psychiatry), one nurse researcher, and three experienced research nurses. We planned to conduct EBP classes in a discussion education format for 30 minutes before day and evening shifts, twice monthly. The sessions included a case study approach to assist staff in (1) generating clinical questions; (2) identifying the sources and levels of evidence; (3) becoming acquainted with the mechanics of a systematic review; and (4) designing EBP interventions. We evaluated incorporating EBP into the identified patient care plan at the end of one cycle. We were watering and nurturing the seedlings.

The garden was planted. We introduced EBP as a process. We taught definition, required steps, and our plan of action. We taught how to query practice and stimulated discussion. The nurses asked, "What is the optimal type and frequency of monitoring to assure patient safety during blood transfusions?" To address this, we conducted a search of vital sign monitoring. Joanna Briggs Institute's systematic review of vital signs was the best resource that provided strong evidence for monitoring. This provoked the nurses to identify more questions specific to blood transfusions, our hospital policy, and our unit practices. They examined current practice and policy. Eventually, nurses became involved in the hospital transfusion committee and implemented policy and procedure changes. More seedlings flourished!

The garden was in bloom! The nurses asked another set of questions: "What are the optimal actions that nurses can take to protect neutropenic patients? Should patients with neutropenia be in private rooms, be admitted to the same unit with patients (in other rooms) who have active infections? Or does this situation pose too great a risk to the neutropenic patient?" All of the nurses were interested; we assisted them in finding and critically appraising the relevant literature. Consequently, the nurses prepared multiple presentations, and their excitement about practice improved. The ground was fertile indeed.

Regarding neutropenia, the nurses also became curious about diet restrictions, pets, and general protection in the hospital environment. Again, we assisted the nurses in finding and critically appraising literature for the best available evidence for low microbial diets for neutropenia. We brought our bounty to the hospital nutrition committee, and the changes were made in the dietary restrictions that are now incorporated into practice.

Another nurse was concerned about pet visitation for these patients. By now the garden path was well worn, the search for evidence was on, and the result was support for a pet policy change for patients with neutropenia. Finally, another question emerged. "What type of masks do neutropenic patients need to wear when out of the room?"

With such plant growth, the garden was growing even more productive. A spirit of inquiry had been ignited, and asking key questions was becoming a regular activity. A new question emerged about the need for fluid restrictions for patients on a medical-surgical unit who also require chronic hemodialysis. Another question involved best management of skin reactions due to radiation therapy. Yet another nurse asked, "Are hydrocolloidal dressings the most effective treatment for wound healing?" Still another question that impacted all of the nurses was whether blood sampling for PT/PTTs were best obtained from central or peripheral lines. After the garden took off, there was no stopping it!

We continued to assist nurses using our available gardening tools: our medical librarian, advanced practice nurses, nurse researcher, nurses with other specialties (e.g., IV nurse clinician, hemodialysis), and medical media department. Presentations became professional, utilizing advanced technology to showcase processes and findings. We assisted nurses with writing abstracts for conferences and coached them on their podium and poster presentations when they were accepted. Our garden needed minimal fertilizer at this point.

By the end of 2005, we evaluated our project using surveys and process notes. Participation involved 10 staff per session, and staff from 2 other hospital units attended. Greater than 50% of staff participated in discussions, greater than 50% of the time the nurse manager participated, and 5 staff presented individual sessions. Staff members were engaged, involved in changing procedures and developing guidelines, and they presented findings at research conferences. Our staff satisfaction survey revealed that 75% of the nurses felt more confident to question practices observed on the unit, 93% felt more confident to make practice changes based on the evidence, 50% were stimulated to think about practice issues but needed support in refining the clinical question, and 100% would recommend to colleagues that they attend an EBP session. The bounty was abundant!

As we presented findings from this project, word spread in the hospital, and other nursing units wanted involvement. The development of journal clubs began. In 2006, we decided to create an EBP subcommittee of the nursing research committee, with Deborah as chair. The members were staff nurse champions of their unit-based journal clubs. We gave initial introductions to EBP and supported these champions in facilitating journal clubs. We formed a special leadership group for these journal club leaders and met frequently to discuss challenges and share successful strategies. So, now we had a Journal Club Facilitators group, an EBP Subcommittee, and a Nursing Research Committee. As the garden grew, the whole look of the neighborhood improved.

Journal club evolution was inspirational. The advanced practice nurse (APN) journal club, in existence since 1993, became recognized as the model. Specialty units, such as oncology, GI, and dialysis, began their own journal clubs. Gradually, up to 15 journal clubs were occurring! We decided we needed a method of evaluation. We needed to learn how to harvest our crop.

Marti tasked a graduate nursing student from the University of San Francisco to evaluate journal clubs—something that had not been done before. Using informal observations and discussions, she categorized her journal club observations according to Everett Rogers' five stages of the adoption of innovations: knowledge, persuasion, decision, implementation, and confirmation. This innovative approach enabled our tool development, now in use with good psychometric properties. A score provides a measure of nurses' perceptions about their professional growth specific to journal clubs. Still more developments have emerged including an EBP Workshop Day in 2008 and the development of Nursing Grand Rounds for EBP project presentations in 2009. Marti and Deborah now cochair the Nursing Research and EBP Council and in 2010 and 2011 classes for EBP and writing are planned.

In conclusion, the seed of one idea has grown into a beautiful, thriving, productive garden. With administrative support, guidance from advanced practice nurses, and use of available resources, our culture change has matured beautifully. The entire process has been inspirational and fun. Best of all, the nurses are staying, and they are knowingly providing our veterans with the best possible care!

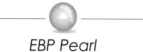

EBP Pearl

It often takes an enthusiastic team to ignite a spirit of inquiry (which is Step 0, and the foundation in the EBP process), and build a culture of evidence-based practice.

From Doctor's Handmaiden to EBP Maven

–*Christine Busch, BSN, RN*
Preoperative Unit
Saint John's Health Center,
Santa Monica, California

My friend and colleague M.B. and I signed up for a mandatory class at work about something called evidence-based practice (EBP). We were not sure what it entailed, but getting paid for 4 hours of education was enticing. We each requested one of the first classes.

I was enthralled with the challenge of research-based care decisions and the concept that bedside nurses could participate in these decisions. I was in nursing school in the 1960s, and no questions or comments were allowed. You did as you were told and taught. I was amazed and excited to learn nursing schools were actually teaching nurses how to engage in EBP.

After class, M.B. spoke at length with our instructor and learned about an annual EBP conference at UCLA. We immediately signed up for the day. We were greeted with rooms full of EBP and research projects by nurses, wonderful speakers, a fabulous lunch, and free pens.

On seeing and hearing our enthusiasm, our instructor offered M.B. and me a chance to apply to the September 2009 EBP Immersion class at Arizona State University College of Nursing and Health Innovation. Our hospital had a grant from UniHealth, which paid for our participation in the weeklong session. Closer to the time we were to depart, we read the e-mail stating that we needed computers and would be required to present a PowerPoint on the last day. Panic ensued!

I had a hand-me-down computer, but I didn't know how to type. M.B. had to borrow a computer the day before we flew out. The instructions we received were talking about program compatibilities. I asked my son if my computer with the apple on it would work.

I rolled into class the first day and watched other participants confidently plug in their computers and set up their desk space. Having supreme observational skills from years of nursing, I quickly followed suit. Most of the nurses in the class had a master's degree, PhD, or experience with EBP projects at their place of employment. This was a plus for me. All were very helpful in answering my questions and helping me learn the technology and terminology. (How do you use a thumb drive without erasing files?) A roomful of teachers graciously helped with thoughtful suggestions and explanations. Tolerant tech support reinforced the positive experience of the week.

The learning curve was steep and rapid. In my experience, nurses are problem solvers. I was determined to complete the project to the best of my ability. I listened intently, asked questions, researched computer help screens, read instructions, went out to eat with new friends from all over the United States, and called M.B. at 2 A.M. as we worked on our presentations. In fact, you could hear my phone calls to her ringing in the background of her final presentation. We were not sure how to erase the ringing without erasing the presentation. My voice-over PowerPoint did not work correctly, and a fellow classmate helped me download my presentation and record it on her computer as the clock was ticking that final morning, an example of the teamwork and support evident throughout the entire week.

Fast forward 11 months, and I have just finished presenting my near-completed research project on preoperative smoking cessation to the nursing director and advanced practice nurses at our hospital. I presented it at Nursing Grand Rounds earlier this year.

M.B. is the coinvestigator. The PhD-prepared instructor of our first introductory EBP class at our hospital is our protocol faculty mentor. The PICOT question is: In preoperative patients (Patient population), how does smoking-cessation educational information via telephone counseling (Intervention of interest) versus no counseling (Comparison intervention) change the time that they decide to smoke their last cigarette (Outcome) preoperatively to 12 hours or greater before scheduled surgery (Time)?

Our preoperative unit typically contacts patients the day before their scheduled surgery. This is the time frame within which we had to work. The data we have collected suggests that telephone counseling can change the time of the last cigarette to 12 hours or greater before the scheduled surgery time. The data collection is complete, and we plan on sending it to the statistician for evaluation. We are discussing making this educational statement a formal part of our preoperative process.

The UniHealth grant for EBP terminated on August 31, 2010. More than 300 nurses completed our hospital EBP course. The hospital professes an ongoing commitment to EBP, although the PhD-prepared instructor is not continuing after the grant termination. I did most of my work on the smoking-cessation project from home because I had no time at work to research articles and review data. In my opinion, this grant was a gift to the hospital that helped jump-start EBP awareness and practice.

After the EBP Mentorship Immersion experience, I became committed to learning how to type with more than two fingers. I received a gift of typing lessons last year, which I have yet to use. I am hopeful that our hospital will make better use of the EBP program "gift" than I have made of my gift. The future has yet to demonstrate how our hospital will continue to benefit from this gift of EBP.

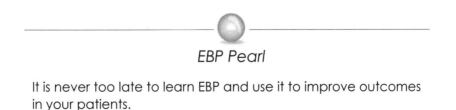

EBP Pearl

It is never too late to learn EBP and use it to improve outcomes in your patients.

Putting the Spirit of Nursing Back Into the Assessment of Labor Pain: The Coping With Labor Algorithm

–Janet Fisher, RNC
Staff Nurse, Labor & Delivery
University of Utah Hospital, Salt Lake City, Utah

–Leissa Roberts, DNP, CNM
Associate Professor (Clinical),
Executive Director of Faculty Practice
University of Utah College of Nursing, Salt Lake City, Utah

–Brenda Gulliver, MS, RN, CNL
Quality Improvement Specialist
University of Utah Hospital, Park City, Utah

We labor nurses and midwives have to quickly connect with our patients and their families in an effort to offer support and encouragement throughout the delivery experience. Although some universals are involved in childbirth, every woman's experience in labor is influenced by her unique social, experiential, and cultural factors. In an effort to understand these influences, we make ongoing assessments to help gain an appreciation of this woman's ability to cope with her labor and birth. The challenge for us is to be adaptive and have the ability to support and champion the woman in whatever childbirth experience she chooses, from an unmedicated delivery to the "How soon can I have my epidural?" approach.

Although one of the most common universals in labor and childbirth is pain, it is not easily defined, nor is it simple to assess. Women describe the sensation of their contractions in a variety of ways, and these sensations can vary in type and intensity as labor progresses. Traditionally, nurses and midwives have ongoing discussions with laboring women about contraction pain and offer options to assist the woman cope with her labor. This time-honored dynamic process was challenged when most hospitals in the United States (US) adopted standardized pain assessments so that they would be in compliance with the Joint Commission's (JC) pain standard, which requires hospitals and other health care facilities to create policies to ensure that (1) their staff are competent to assess pain, and (2) all patients have their pain assessed on an ongoing basis.

After the JC's standard was published, our hospital adopted the numeric rating scale (NRS) as the standardized method for pain assessment, which is one of the most commonly used, reliable and established pain assessments in the US. Soon after implementing the NRS for pain assessment, the labor and delivery (L&D) staff expressed dissatisfaction with the effectiveness of this tool to assess labor pain. The staff felt that instead of conveying a sense of concern and an intent to help women manage their labor, most patients were confused and/or annoyed by the nurses' ongoing request for them to "rate" their current level of pain. Our nursing staff identified that NRS pain assessment did not allow for the progressive nature of labor pain.

That realization led to the creation of a task force to investigate if another way would meet our patients' needs and meet the requirements of the JC standard and our hospital's policy. The task force comprised experienced L&D nurses and a faculty member from the local college of nursing, nurse midwifery program.

An assistant professor at the University of Utah's College of Nursing was one of the authors of the Joint Commission's pain standard. She agreed to meet with the leader of our task force to clarify the intent of the JC standard, and she made us aware of the following statement in the standard: "If applicable, separate specialized assessment and reassessment information is identified for the various populations served." Gaining an appreciation of this piece of the standard excited the task force. We naively thought that if we went to the "powers that be" at the hospital and told them that the NRS didn't work for our patient population, they would allow us to go back to our time-honored (but undefined) methods of assessing labor pain.

Though we knew the nurses were dissatisfied with the NRS process, we didn't have concrete information about the patients' responses to the scale, so our next step was to gather data to gain insight into the patient perspective. We interviewed a sample of postpartum patients who had vaginal deliveries and found two common themes: first, they stated confusion about when they should rate pain (with contractions or in between contractions), and secondly, patients complained about the nurses' ongoing requests for them to rate their pain. These findings from our internal evidence survey corroborated our anecdotal conclusions.

The task force felt we were now ready to make our case to the hospital's pain improvement group. We made an impassioned argument, but instead of the hoped-for release from having to use the NRS pain assessment tool and permission to return to our old time-honored methods, we were directed to find and present more data as we searched for an evidence-based (not time-honored) alternative method. Little did we know at the time that we were starting the process of developing a new pain assessment tool for laboring women.

The task force approached this challenge as a quality improvement project. We searched the literature and found hardly any evidence about managing labor pain. We found that the two authors who wrote specifically about assessing labor pain encouraged the use of open-ended questions with such terms as *coping* and *comfort*. After long discussions about the implication of these two words, the group settled on *coping* as a more accurate descriptor of how we saw women working through their labor process. Settling on a common term to use to describe the phenomenon led us to frame "coping questions" that would assist the nurse in the assessment of labor pain. The development of these questions enabled task force members to discuss the whole concept of pain management of the laboring woman. During these task force pain revisioning sessions, we started to map out various nonpharmacological and pharmacological approaches that the collective *we* had effectively used when caring for women in labor (i.e., gathering internal evidence). Members of the task force were pretty fired up about the discovery process we were in, and many took this discussion out to the rest of the staff. Most of the staff became engaged in this conversation, and not only were more contributions made to the algorithm we were creating, but also many staff tried out new techniques with their patients and then shared their experiences. The dynamic process led to an all-inclusive diagram that we called the Coping with Labor Algorithm. The algorithm generated many clinical questions so that in time we sought out and evaluated the evidence for all of nonpharmacologic methods listed in the algorithm.

When the task force finished the draft of the Coping with Labor Algorithm, it represented most of the time-honored methods. However, those traditions were now in an organized format that not only promoted use of open-ended coping questions in assessing labor pain, but also described and directed the nurse on many of the other options available to assist a woman to cope with her labor. Practical application of the algorithm was then put to the test with a series of in-house implementations. Modifications to the algorithm were made based on the staff's experience with using it. Data from these algorithm implementations was gathered and presented to the hospital's pain improvement group. After reviewing the information, this authority agreed that the Coping with Labor Algorithm be the sole method of pain assessment in labor.

The staff were elated by the pain improvement group's decision and felt pride in their participation in the process of developing an assessment that worked for us and the women for whom we care. It opened our eyes to question and to believe that staff nurses can develop and promote best practices. The algorithm now has become a teaching tool for novice L&D nurses. We felt our pain assessment tool was very effective for assessing pain in labor, but we were not sure how the Joint Commission would view our innovation. During our next JC survey, the chart of a laboring woman was scrutinized by a surveyor, and during the general debrief, the surveyors made a comment that the staff was *consistent and correct* in pain assessment.

Since this important work, two journal articles have been published about the Coping with Labor Algorithm. The first described the process undertaken to develop and implement the algorithm; the other identifies the level of evidence for the interventions listed under the nonpharmacological branch of the algorithm. As a result of these publications, we received an overwhelmingly positive response from both the national and international L&D nurse and midwife community. To date, we have received hundreds of inquiries about the algorithm. The Coping with Labor Algorithm also has been translated into several languages. Furthermore, we did a telepresentation for the IHI Perinatal Community. Not only did this evidence-based project have an impact on the experience of labor for women, but we, as L&D nurses, felt much more in control of our practice.

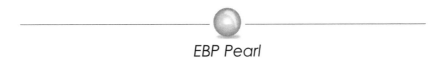

EBP Pearl

Evidence-based clinicians always question the status quo, but don't throw the baby out with the bathwater!

Conscience Perceptions

–JoAnn Franklin, DNP, RN
Doctor of Nursing Practice Program Candidate
Saint Louis University School of Nursing, Potosi, Missouri

Caring for patients in Urgent Care was sometimes routine and sometimes a challenge, but my approach during my 6 years of working there was always the same—to give care to all patients as though they were my own family. The night I saw this 82-year-old man was no exception. He actually was the grandfather of a hospital medical floor nurse named Lisa.

This elderly man presented with a chief complaint of "flu." I went in the exam room with my thoughts collected on giving care for influenza. I always try to formulate a plan by reviewing the chart before seeing the patient. I have found out over the years that it does not always work out as planned because many times the complaint given in triage is not really the reason patients provide for me when asked why they are in Urgent Care.

This night the complaint remained the same; he believed he had the flu. This elderly, frail man was surrounded by his children and grandchildren, who all were there to get him treatment for his flu. I always do a thorough history and physical exam, and this night was no different. Lisa's grandpa was sick. The family was concerned that he just was not able to shake it and appeared to be getting worse. Everyone seemed concerned that he was lethargic and *not himself.*

I gathered information and began examining Grandpa with a focus on his respiratory exam, which all family present resoundingly indicated was his reason for being at the clinic. In the process of my exam, I noticed bruising on his arm, and upon further questioning and investigation, found that this gentleman reported experiencing several falls over the last few days, including one striking his head on the corner of the kitchen table. He had no explanation for the cause of these falls and had no prior history of falls. His head showed no evidence of trauma on exam. Grandpa's exam basically demonstrated respiratory findings of wheezing and a cough with a low grade temperature. The rest was a normal exam, including his neurological exam, but things seemed unusual. My clinical expertise kicked in, and I decided that the report of a head injury warranted a computerized axial tomography (CT) of the head. The bruising on his arm was mild, but

Grandpa's mental status changes required a comprehensive workup, despite the fact that these were not part of his complaint. The standard of care indicated a head CT be done because of the mental status changes and a recent head injury. Lisa's grandpa was thoroughly assessed and had appropriate testing.

Soon after Lisa's grandpa returned to his exam room after completing his head CT, the radiologist called with his report—bilateral subdural hematomas. The radiologist explained that having bilateral hematomas equalized the neurological exam so that grandpa exhibited no neurological findings of a subdural hematoma except for the fatigue and subtle, mild mental status changes that his family attributed to Grandpa having the flu.

The family was shocked to learn Grandpa would be flown by helicopter to a larger St. Louis hospital with a neurosurgery specialty for treatment of his hematomas. They gathered in amazement thinking that a flu had been the reason that grandpa was *not himself* and that he had not been able to *shake the bug*. The family was grateful that their loved one was diagnosed and on his way to treatment for his traumatic head injury.

I was thanking my clinical expertise—thoroughness, conscience perception, and instinct—for not missing a critical finding that could have ended in Grandpa's demise. Following evidence provided by the patient's history and exam, practicing with skill, and taking time to listen, look, and gather subtle clues (i.e., evidence-based practice) can save lives. Not asking questions and focusing only on the *flu* would have had serious consequences. Holistic, evidence-based care delivery gave me the ability to recognize more than a chief complaint; it allowed me to look beyond the complaint of *flu* and see Lisa's grandpa as a whole person with complex needs, not just an illness. Grandpa's neurosurgery went well and resulted in a full recovery with a return to his loving family.

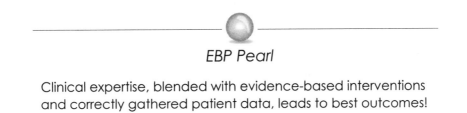

EBP Pearl

Clinical expertise, blended with evidence-based interventions and correctly gathered patient data, leads to best outcomes!

Passion Rekindled With Evidence-Based Practice

–Dianna D. Inman, DNP, APRN, CPNP-PC
Assistant Professor
University of North Carolina at Charlotte,
Charlotte, North Carolina

As I reflect on my career as a nurse and an advanced practice nurse, I realized that it was not about patient care anymore; it was about the bottom line—money. I was practicing in a specialty outpatient clinic at a major university. There it became apparent that the majority of our discussions in clinic meetings revolved around billing issues, and seldom, if at all, did we talk about patient outcomes. I would spend several hours with the patient and family and then write a six-page comprehensive note regarding that visit, including a laundry list of recommendations, to no avail. The majority of the time, the patient and family returned, having initiated none of the interventions I recommended.

Then, I had the opportunity to move my practice into a school-based clinic. There I had immediate access to the students, families, and teachers. It was not long before I recognized that the current model of care that I had been taught in the university-based clinic would not meet the needs of the students at this school. The students and families' needs at this high-risk school were great. When I considered that, combined with the limited resources and funding, I knew the only approach that could possibly address issues was evidence-based practice. In my Doctor of Nursing Practice program, I was taught to identify the problem in my clinical setting, search the literature, and formulate a plan based on the evidence, implement the plan, and evaluate its effectiveness. Not only did I focus on the individual patient and problem, but I could also look broader at the issues causing the problem. The evidence revealed that early prevention was the key to addressing the majority of the issues that affected my patients and families.

Evidence-based interventions were tailored to the school and the community. Student suspension rates and referrals to the office decreased, and classroom atmosphere saw an overall improvement. This renewed my belief that we can make a difference when we look at practice from a broader perspective and use the evidence to address the most challenging problems that face children and families of this nation. At the end of the day, it is not about the number of patients that we see, but about making the best clinical decision based on the most current evidence that will have a lasting effect on our patients.

Evidence-based practice renewed my passion to provide the best possible care at a time in my career where I saw priorities of care shifting from quality to quantity of care.

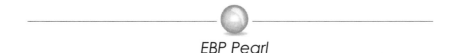

EBP Pearl

EBP makes a difference for patients, yes, and it makes a difference for providers!

The Moisture Chamber: A Journey Into Evidence-Based Practice

–*Kerri Jones, BS, RN*
Nurse Clinician II-M, Department of Neuroscience Nursing
The Johns Hopkins Hospital, Baltimore, Maryland

As a relatively new nurse, I was naive to the concept of evidence-based practice (EBP). Needless to say, when I was scheduled for a departmental evidence-based project workshop, I was both excited and puzzled. I had limited exposure to the concept of EBP in nursing school—although as any nurse can attest, nursing school is a retrospective blur. Nonetheless, this scheduled workshop piqued my interest, and I anxiously awaited its time.

The first day of the workshop arrived, and I sat surrounded by a group of eight of my peers, most of whom I had seen around the department and many I knew to be more senior than me. The instructors arrived. They encompassed a range of expertise including the assistant director of neuroscience nursing and the neuroscience nurse educator.

"What is EBP?" That is what I came to find out, and that is the question that set me off on a journey of education, practice evaluation, and in the end, practice justification. Day one was filled with getting answers. What is EBP? What is involved in the EBP process? Most importantly, how does this apply to me? Our group quickly learned that EBP was something we used every day, a basis for our profession. EBP values current evidence-based nursing treatments and procedures, and incorporates current research in future care interventions. Using quality research when it is available or conducting research when the evidence does not exist should be the pinnacle of every evolving health profession, especially nursing.

After learning the ins and outs of EBP, my group and I brainstormed ideas for an evidence-based project. What in our everyday practice had no clear definition of the "why" behind it? What task did we perform regularly with no other reason than because it was ordered by the medical team? In this brainstorming, we were quick to realize that many treatments we performed were simply done because "that's how it was always done," with no clear, current research-based reasoning behind it. Narrowing down the topics, we finally agreed upon one: the moisture chamber.

In the department of neuroscience, the moisture chamber is used following a craniotomy to help keep the eye injury-free in the presence of a cranial nerve deficit. We all knew what it was, but none of us knew where the idea came from. Additionally, none of us knew if the treatment of the moisture chamber was even the best practice indicated for postcraniotomy patients with cranial nerve palsy.

We had a topic for our project, but now where did we begin? The second part of the workshop was filled with searching for evidence to address the clinical issue. After determining the different ways to conduct a search for the evidence, off to the library we went to explore the vast resources available to us. A librarian from the Welch Medical Library walked us through a step-by-step scavenger hunt of information available on our topic. The sheer amount of resources we were exposed to was enough to leave all of our heads spinning. Like kids in a candy store, we sat at our terminals gathering article after article based on our question about the moisture chamber. Then it was back to the conference where we could critically appraise our evidence and devise a plan to gather internal evidence from practice data.

We systematically evaluated each article we obtained from the evidence search, critically appraising for both strength and quality. Next, we assigned the task of seeking expert testimony from the department's practicing neurosurgeons, as well as the hospital's ophthalmology department. Additionally, some group members were assigned the task of contacting comparable hospitals to gather benchmark data; that is, to obtain their standards of practice and outcomes for using the moisture chamber. At the close of the second week, we were hopeful that when we met again, we would have appropriate internal and external evidence to support the practice of the moisture chamber.

At our last meeting, we brought all of our hard work together. We had current, applicable research supporting the use of the moisture chamber. In addition, we had supportive testimony from experts in the field as well as comparative practice data (internal evidence) from the nation's other leading medical institutions. All of this was impressive—we had actually substantiated with evidence a task we perform every day. We could now, with certainty, conclude that the moisture chamber was the best practice. This was a career-altering event for me. I realized that every undertaking in my profession, every procedure I perform with a patient, comes from more than an order written on a chart. This notion was exhilarating.

To wrap up, in the EBP workshop, we discussed evidence-based protocols. Having just established best care with our evidence, it was time to substantiate it through writing a standard of care that every patient who met the criteria for the moisture chamber would receive. As a direct result of our project, an addendum to the Management of the Postoperative Neurosurgical Patient Protocol was created to include the moisture chamber as a standard of care.

The EBP workshop changed my professional life. I find myself often contemplating the "whys" of my profession. Each procedure/treatment I perform has taken on a new shade of legitimacy. A sense of accomplishment comes to me every time I review the postop protocol and see the moisture chamber addition. I have a smile of satisfaction knowing that nursing is a profession supported and surrounded by the best available research and internal evidence.

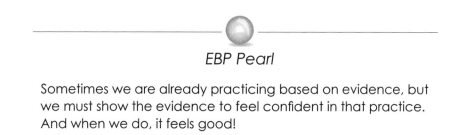

EBP Pearl

Sometimes we are already practicing based on evidence, but we must show the evidence to feel confident in that practice. And when we do, it feels good!

In Charge of Your Unit as Well as Your Career

–Susan McInerney, BSN, RN, CPN
Charge Nurse
St. Christopher's Hospital for Children,
Philadelphia, Pennsylvania

I've witnessed many changes throughout my nursing career—most good; however, some are best left in the past. Having graduated from nursing school in 1984, I have practiced bedside nursing following various models of care such as team nursing, primary nursing, and random assignment nursing. I've worked in pediatrics on both critical care and general med-surg nursing units. Approximately 7 years ago, our hospital started on the journey toward Magnet designation. In doing so, the hospital implemented many changes to drive us toward our goal. Having graduated before the process of evidence-based practice (EBP) existed as part of nursing school curriculum, let alone as part of the average bedside nurse's vocabulary and practice, I was interested and uncertain about what to expect. I thought "What is EBP anyway, and how will I, a nurse of 20-plus years of experience, learn and adjust? I'll let the newer graduate nurses do this. After all, they just learned about it in school. I'll just keep doing what I have always been doing." Fortunately for me, our nursing leadership recognized this as a real challenge that would need to be overcome. They provided information about EBP tools and education to all involved in patient care, including their "seasoned nurses." Upon learning about EBP, I realized that our practice would be challenged and require improvement, but some areas would remain unchanged as they were already evidence-based.

The most significant and personal EBP experience for me was the creation of the permanent charge nurse role. This role was developed as an EBP initiative spearheaded by a group of staff nurses who were supported by our hospital's nursing leadership. This meant that the charge nurse role and responsibilities would no longer be randomly assigned to the most experienced nurse or the nurse who volunteered that day to be in charge while still shouldering a full patient-care assignment. The charge nurse role is a budgeted position, which enables the person hired specifically for that role to be identified as point person on their shift for physicians, services, and departments. In my role as charge nurse, I can support our nurses as they need during their shift. This role enables me to perform daily rounding with patients and families so that issues can be addressed early. I work with our unit's shared governance council to target specific patient and staff satisfaction areas that then have a positive impact on our scores. With all hospitals facing economic challenges, as the charge nurse I can devote significant attention to maximizing shift staffing patterns, which can impact our unit's budget.

These aspects of my charge nurse role occur on a daily basis; however, I also have been able to get involved in professional poster development and presentations at outside conferences. Most recently, as a member of our research council, I was involved in the development of an EBP presentation to our nursing department, truly a full circle moment. I was delighted when I was asked by our chief nursing officer to attend the national Magnet conference as a representative from our hospital. I clearly remember sitting on the plane and thinking, "I can't believe I am on this plane flying to this national conference. Who would have ever thought, after all these years, a staff nurse would have these opportunities." My nursing career has not only been reenergized, but redefined in a way that keeps evolving beyond what I could have ever envisioned before we started on our Magnet journey.

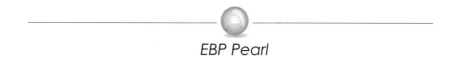

EBP Pearl

Simple evidence-based solutions bring remarkable rewards!

Saying Goodbye to the Sacred Cows in the Operating Room

–Ellice Mellinger, MS, RN, CNOR
Clinical Nurse Educator for Perioperative Services
University Medical Center, Tucson, Arizona

I have been a perioperative nurse for over 30 years. I personally have been on some exciting adventures as the evidence-based nursing practice (EBNP) movement has changed nursing practice in our institution. I started my career as a medical-surgical

RN on a respiratory care unit, and then I went into the operating room (OR). I worked many years as an OR staff RN. Currently, I am a clinical nurse educator in a university medical center. I have always liked the science of nursing. My mother, who was an RN diploma grad from the 1940s, always teased me and called me her "BS" nurse—I don't think she was referring to "bachelor of science"!

When I first started in the operating room, I would ask "why" questions that would many times be answered with "because we have always done it this way"; "because that is what the doctor ordered"; or "I really don't know." One example of a "sacred cow," or traditional practice, that I remember most clearly is this: I was taught to perform preoperative skin preps for the surgical patient and vary the time of the skin prep procedure because of the location of the incision. We used to prep the patient's abdomen for 5 minutes and prep the patient's knees, hip, and head for 10 minutes. I was told that we did this because if a patient having orthopedic or neurosurgery gets an infection, it is "a lot worse" for them. I don't remember reading about the evidence to support this practice.

Back then, not many of my nurse colleagues spoke about the "nursing research" or "the evidence" to support nursing practices. Soon after I started working in the operating room, I joined a national organization, the Association of Operating Room Nurses (AORN), which has now evolved to the Association of PeriOperative Nurses. Through this organization (and my mentor nurses who were interested in the "whys"), I learned about national nursing standards and recommended practices for the surgical patient. I think many of the standards and recommended practices were a consensus of best practices from experienced OR nurses who participated in national committees to write them. I know now that the opinions of the expert nurse are valuable, and these continue to contribute to EBNP, but I don't know how much evidence was available to support their practices.

About 6 years ago, I attended a seminar about evidence-based nursing practice at our medical center. Our medical center was beginning to introduce the concept of EBNP to our nurses. All of our OR nurses, new and not so new, attended the class, and we were all very excited about EBNP. We came up with an idea to incorporate an EBNP project into the operating room RN internship program, which was supported by the leadership team. To facilitate the project, I worked with our committee chair of nursing research, and can report that for the past 5 years, we have had a process in place for our new nurses in the perioperative areas to work on EBNP issues.

The nurses in the OR and the post-anesthesia care unit (PACU) RN internship programs have time away from the unit to work on these projects. The nurses have a specific timeline, specific guidelines to follow, and are mentored by other resource persons and me in the medical center. The nurses select a topic of interest in perioperative nursing and follow the EBNP checklist we developed. Part of the requirement to complete the project includes the nurse presenting his or her findings at the respective staff meetings. As part of the project, a slide presentation is created that tells about the project and is placed on our intranet as a reference for all medical center staff members.

As a result of these EBNP projects, I believe our nurses have grown in their professional careers. The nurses have questioned current protocols and policies and have searched to find best practices about a variety of nursing topics. For example, one of our OR nurses wanted to find the best practices to prevent venous thromboembolism in the surgical patient. As a result of her work, a nursing protocol was developed, and she was asked to present her EBNP project at a national nursing conference. As a result of this kind of EBNP project, I believe our patients have benefited from changes in patient care, and nursing protocols have been updated and improved.

On a personal note, I have grown in my career because of my work with developing the EBNP project program and mentoring nurses. An initial example of that would be when my colleague and I submitted an abstract to a local nursing conference that was accepted, thereby enabling us to present to our community the ideas that had so helped our nurses and patients. Since then, I have presented poster and podium presentations at local, regional, and national nursing conferences about the EBNP project work that brought me national recognition from AORN. I was honored to be the recipient of the national AORN Outstanding Achievement in Perioperative Evidence-Based Practice Award. Furthermore, I have recently been asked to write an article about our projects for the *AORN Journal* as a guest editorial. These opportunities would not likely have happened to me without EBNP.

I think the EBNP movement is helping us weed out the sacred cows so we can question everyday nursing practices. EBNP reminds us as nurses that inquiry is important to our work, and we need to practice nursing with the current best evidence to help our patients achieve their best outcomes. Because of EBNP, my nursing practice and my nursing career have provided me with rich opportunities and experiences. I know this would make my mother proud.

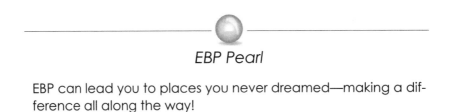

EBP Pearl

EBP can lead you to places you never dreamed—making a difference all along the way!

Evidence-Based Practice: A Way of Life

–Kathleen Pecoraro, BSN, RN, CPAN
Staff nurse
Northern Westchester Hospital,
Mt. Kisco, New York

I went to nursing school in the early 1980s. At that time, nothing resembling EBP was taught. Long before I heard the term "evidence-based practice" (EBP), I questioned, "Why am I doing what I do?" EBP is a thought process for me, a way of life. As I grew as a nurse, I began to question "why *we* do the things *we* do." I questioned not only clinical issues, but professional issues as well. For example, "back in the day," nurses gave up their chairs to physicians. Why did we need to do that? We were mostly women—aka ladies! The physicians were, of course, mostly men. Another issue that I questioned was why must we wear only white? I have always felt that white is quite an impractical color to wear, even though I really like to wear a white T-shirt with my jeans. White is impractical not only because of the blood and body fluids we inadvertently smeared on ourselves, but also because of the coffee stains and pen marks. All of my white clothing quickly became quite stained. I am happy to report that I am now able to wear different colors to work as a staff nurse.

Over the past 2 years, Northern Westchester Hospital (NWH) has implemented a program of shared governance. I belong to the EBP/Nursing Research Council. Learning about EBP has been interesting and exciting to me. The EBP process is very much like the nursing process. Both are scientific, concrete, defined, and measurable. I love facts I can hold on to. I find myself asking "why" questions more often. For example, I wondered, "Why is our blanket warmer only at 110 degrees Fahrenheit, when it had been up to 130 degrees 6 months ago?" Our postoperative patients loved the very warm blankets. More questions that occurred—How far should a foley be inserted before inflating the balloon? Why was a policy written a certain way? Is there evidence to back up what is written in the policy? Questions like these can be answered by searching for their answers in different databases and, of course, by asking more questions. I love the investigative aspect of EBP. You never know where a question or project might take you! Answering questions gives a sense of professional empowerment that comes from becoming the expert on a subject I find interesting.

I have been a staff nurse for 28 years. Over the years, at times it has been discouraging to witness certain trends in nursing. I believe nurses generally feel they do not have a voice pertaining to issues that are important to them, particularly as staff nurses. Learning, living, practicing, making mistakes, and learning even more has renewed my nursing spirit. I have a voice, thanks to the framework of EBP. I do not want to change the world; I am interested in improving my patients' outcomes. But by working on improving our patients' outcomes, we can make a change in the world, however large or small that change might be. Since becoming involved with, living, and learning EBP, I view myself as a staff nurse with the heart of a nursing scientist—something that I feel deep within my gut.

Some people within any organization want to keep things just as they always have been, want to maintain the "status quo." I have run into just this issue within my organization. Persons higher up the "food chain" than I were providing misinformation about a subject that I was investigating. Well, in EBP, opinions of respected authorities are lower level evidence. I did my "EBP thing," searched the data bases for higher level evidence, and found the evidence supported what I was seeking to do. Fortunately, many people within the organization are supportive of best practice, supportive of the acquisition of new knowledge and ideas, and these persons gladly support me.

As a post-anesthesia care unit (PACU) nurse, the only large project I have worked on and completed (so far!) involved normothermia in surgical patients. The National Surgical Care Improvement Project (SCIP) identified hypothermia in general and spinal anesthesia patients as a risk factor for postoperative (postop) infections, as well as other postop complications. NWH's quality dashboard identified a high percentage of hypothermic postoperative patients. The surgical services director asked the EBP representatives to work on fixing this problem.

The operating room (OR) EBP representative, Wendy, and I began working together on this venture. Fay, our mentor on the EBP/Nursing Research Council, provided support throughout the process. As time passed, SCIP dropped the specific normothermia requirement and merely required measures be taken to prevent hypothermia in the OR. The intervention we chose to institute in our OR was to keep the OR ambient temperature between 68–72 degrees Fahrenheit until the "time-out" procedure, at which point the patient is completely covered. Then, the room temperature can be adjusted to staff comfort. As it turned out, Diane and Eunice, our OR educators, were in need of a clinical competency for this year. We collaborated on the development of the clinical competency. This competency has helped to facilitate sustainability for this practice change. Simple monitoring of outcomes also helps ensure the practice change continues to be implemented. The surgical services director and I worked with the OR manager to ensure that postoperative temperatures were measured quarterly. Through this project, I gained professional colleagues and personal friends, like Wendy. We have fun at work and enjoyed working together on our normothermia project.

I truly appreciate that EBP gives nurses the ability to provide thoughtful, up-to-date care for patients. Nurses can and have an obligation to ask thoughtful questions and seek the answers. We do not have to continue to do anything because "that is the way it is always done." Nurses are intelligent professionals. Our focus, no matter our specialty, is to provide the best care possible to the patients we serve. By utilizing the EBP framework, we can do just that.

EBP Pearl

"We've always done it that way" is not a viable option for health care in the 21st century!

Revolution of the Mind

–Connie Poon, BSN, RN, CPON
Bone Marrow Transplant Unit
Texas Children's Hospital, Houston, Texas

Most nurses have an innate desire to do the right thing for the patients. The questions are these: How do we know that it is the right thing and where is the source of the information? These were questions I did not ask very often before the evidence-based practice (EBP) course. My main resource for information was from more experienced nurses. I enrolled in the EBP class at Texas Children's Hospital in the fall of 2005. Little did I know at the time that my practice and my view of the nursing profession would be deeply impacted.

My class assignment was to review the nursing policy on *Safe and Effective Use of Aerosolized Ribavirin*. As I went through the process of searching for and analyzing the evidence, I felt like I was just touching the tip of the EBP iceberg. Based on findings from the evidence, stakeholders' insight, and benchmarking results, we recommended a few changes to the nursing policy. Those changes were approved, and the nurses were subsequently educated on the practice change through one of the internal online trainings. For the very first time, I felt I could actually impact nursing practice beyond good bedside care! Knowledge is powerful!

The lessons learned in the EBP class paved the way for many things I did on my own unit and in the hospital. A colleague, who was also an EBP Scholar, and I did a project focused on improving patient compliance with skin and oral hygiene on the bone marrow transplant unit. We wanted to change the occurrence of opportunistic infections in a severely immunocompromised population. We used research findings to demonstrate bacterial growth on skin and in the mouths of these patients. We also used external evidence (research) to substantiate the importance of the use of chlorohexidine in baths and as oral rinses to decrease colonization of *Staphylococcus aureus*. We identified barriers and rallied support from stakeholders. With the findings, we developed education materials for staff, patients, and parents. As a result, the patient compliance rate increased from 40–50% to 85–90%. Again, EBP boosted my confidence about how I could impact practice improvement in my own clinical setting.

Texas Children's Hospital has shared governance councils, namely Clinical Practice, Quality Outcomes and Research, Staff Operations, and Education. As a staff nurse, I have had the opportunity to chair the Clinical Practice Council and to be involved in the EBP Committee. Texas Children's Hospital uses EBP not only as a foundation for policies, protocols, and clinical guidelines, but also for the development of new programs and evaluation of products. Examples of new programs and product evaluations are a) the implementation of procedural pain protocol, b) Demerol precautions, c) a rapid response team, d) an acute chest protocol for sickle cell patients, e) a palliative care team, and f) the securing of devices for peripheral IVs, just to name a few.

On a personal level, EBP revolutionized my way of thinking. I often find myself asking, "Why do I do what I do?" The passion to pursue sound rationale leads to a higher level of critical analysis of nursing interventions and to the engagement of critical dialogue with colleagues and physicians. When I come across conflicting information or need guidance, I try to refer to the policies or guidelines. It is very comforting to know that the nursing policies and clinical guidelines at my institution are based on research evidence. Whether EBP is utilized on a grand institutional scale or at unit level, when evidence is used to shape our practice and decisions, it raises the standard of care; eliminates opinions ruled by popularity, tradition, or habit; ensures consistency among nurses; and promotes a culture of change for the benefit of patient outcome.

EBP Pearl

EBP starts and ends with how you think about your practice!

Stroke Rehabilitation's Team Approach to Reducing Urinary Catheter Infections: Our Evidence-Based Practice Journey

–Sylvia Sanderson, RN
MetroHealth Medical Center
Cleveland, Ohio

Several years ago, I was looking for an opportunity for professional growth because I had been a rehabilitation nurse for over 20 years and felt I wanted to step out of my comfort zone. The hospital in which I work had a wonderful program that allows nurses to advance professionally while remaining at the bedside. The track that I was most interested in was the Evidence-based Practice (EBP) Champion. Within this role, I would have the opportunity to promote and provide quality care by implementing best practices based on evidence in the literature. I decided to apply for the position and soon after became very active in this role on my unit.

My first project involved looking at our present practice around the use of urinary catheters. In October of 2008, I noticed a spike in bladder infection rates on the stroke rehabilitation unit. It seemed like many of the patients with urinary catheters had an infection. First, I pulled together a group of staff to look further into this issue. This included nurses on our practice committee, the unit manager, and physicians. I started to collect data to reflect the incidence of infection, which would give us baseline information about this problem. We knew that infections had an impact on our patients' length of stay, comfort, and how well they performed in therapy. It also can add significantly to the cost of their stay and can affect reimbursement if an infection developed during their stay.

Many of our patients are admitted to our unit, either from within our hospital or as a transfer from other hospitals, with a urinary catheter. Our routine had been to remove the catheter after the patient had experienced several episodes of bowel continence and was able to communicate their need to have a bowel movement. In gathering data about this problem, I found that the urinary catheter puts a patient at higher risk of developing an infection. But what other factors were also involved? Was it a technique/catheter care issue that needed to be addressed? We do switch the larger drainage bags over each day to a smaller, more portable bag they can use while in therapy. As the EBP Champion for our unit, I did a search for evidence to find articles addressing meatal care and aseptic technique. After I obtained the best practice, I provided inservices for all staff so that technique with equipment and solutions used were consistent. Also, I searched for and found studies that supported the use of catheter-securing devices in decreasing the incidence of infections. Based on the evidence, we added catheter-securing devices to our stock of equipment and began using them.

Another factor for this population was the impact of fluid intake on development of infections. We wondered, "Are our patients getting sufficient fluids to flush out their bladders?" Many stroke patients have swallowing issues requiring them to be restricted to thickened fluids. They might simply need a great deal of encouragement and coaxing to take fluids. I wondered, "And what about those fluids?" I found studies in nursing journals that supported simply offering cranberry juice several times a day as effective in reducing the incidence of bladder infections. In addition, many stroke patients have lost strength/dexterity on one side of their body, which makes it difficult to pour water from a pitcher into a glass. We did some problem solving, and came up with the idea of sport bottles with straws instead of water pitchers that the patients could not only use at the bedside, but also take with them to their therapy sessions to increase their fluid intake. We also purchased sip cups with handles and a lid for shaky hands, which many patients found to be helpful.

In reviewing the evidence in nursing and health, the bottom line was that the risk factor that was *most* likely to increase the risk of a patient developing a bladder infection was simply having a urinary catheter. The longer the catheter was in place, the greater chance of developing an infection—period! The evidence was strong, consistent, and compelling. So our nursing team looked at our bladder management protocol. What if we didn't consider bowel continence in determining when to remove the catheter, but rather removed the catheter on admission, unless the patient met certain criteria for keeping the catheter in based on the evidence? Could we change the protocol and get the catheters out much sooner? We chose to change the protocol and put our action plan in place.

Soon after, with support from the physicians, we put our action plan into place. Patients with catheters who needed them because of a urinary retention or other medical reason maintained the catheter with appropriate catheter care and aseptic technique when switching the bags over for therapies. We used a device to secure the tube to the leg to prevent traction or pulling on the catheter tube or displacement. Fluids were monitored, and sport bottles became very popular for the patients—and they took them to therapy. We offered their meds with cranberry juice if they liked it or offered it at bedtime. Patients were assessed for appropriateness of urinary catheters, resulting in many of the catheters being removed much sooner. We were fortunate to have a bladder scanner purchased for the rehabilitation units. This is a terrific noninvasive method to check patients postvoid residuals and can limit reintroducing bacteria into the bladder.

How effective was our team's initiative in reducing bladder infections overall? Well, the numbers tell the story. From October to August the following year, our nosocomial urinary tract infection (UTI) rate dropped by more than 50%! With efforts from all of our team members, this evidence-based performance improvement project made a big difference.

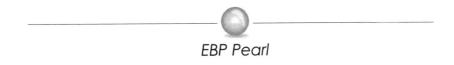

EBP Pearl

Persist in finding the evidence—because evidence rocks!

Changing a Frame of Mind: Skeptic to Believer

–Carol Selby, RN, MT (ASCP)
Infection Prevention
Franklin Square Hospital,
Baltimore, Maryland

At first, I was very skeptical about participating in an evidence-based practice (EBP) project. I worked full-time in the Infection Prevention Department. At the time, I was fairly new to the role, and we were short staffed. Additionally, I was taking classes for my RN to MS degree, and I had never participated in an EBP project before. These activities were on top of my personal life and responsibilities. With all of those reasons, why on earth would I want to put more on my plate? What did capture my attention was a project topic that interested me: evaluating the appropriateness for the insertion of an indwelling urinary catheter. This project would be directly related to my work in the infection prevention department. I spoke to the clinical nurse specialist for evidence-based practice and research at my facility and expressed interest under the condition that I could be partnered with someone on the project.

Then, the process began. I was paired with a medical-surgical nurse with expertise in wound care, Kathy, who shared the same interest. We submitted a formal application for the EBP Internship, which was reviewed by our peers in a blind review process. We were thrilled and honored to be accepted as 2010 EBP Interns at our hospital. As we progressed, working well together, we became great friends. At times, it did feel as though digging through the research was endless. We continued to narrow our evidence using our PICOT question, always staying focused on insertion of the urinary catheter and staying away from the temptation to follow the trail of research for removal of urinary catheters. Kathy and I worked independently to search for and critically appraise the evidence. After forming our own rating of the evidence, we would come together and compare our findings. We critically appraised the articles using the level and quality of evidence adapted from the University of Colorado and using the Iowa model, which we found to be a very straightforward and helpful tool. When we initially started, we had the luxury of a team approach which included other nurses working on EBP projects and our adviser, the clinical nurse specialist for evidence-based practice and research. We would share the articles we wanted to discuss and appraise and then meet to get the group's input. This approach proved to be a great learning experience for the entire group. As time went on and our confidence grew, we found ourselves relying less on the group. The tool gave us the format for rating the level, quality, and type of evidence. We rarely found ourselves in disagreement when we compared our work. If we did have a disagreement, it was very easily resolved by going to the tool and discussing the points together.

We are very fortunate to have a rich base of mentors to draw from at our facility. The clinical nurse specialist for evidence-vased practice and research was the backbone of the process; she was just a phone call or a computer click away. She conducted educational workshops to assist in every step, guiding and at times pushing us to reach our full potential. The medical librarian and her staff were extremely helpful and patient with us in our literature searches. This was one step that has been troublesome and confusing. I feel, as nurses, we don't always have the time, knowledge of, or patience to get the full use of the electronic aids we have available. This experience has definitely helped me to understand how powerful a resource the medical librarian and her staff are in identifying and retrieving literature. I plan to continue to delve into and explore the databases available with the hope of increasing the confidence level that being an EBP intern has created. As a student, the skills to research topics more thoroughly and with better accuracy contribute dramatically to my level of learning. I feel I have just scratched the surface, and I look forward to new opportunities to explore research topics.

I found EBP to be more than translating research or improving outcomes; it truly supports the professional spirit of a nurse. I am very fortunate to be partnered with a staff nurse that had direct patient care, which I lacked, because I am currently working in infection prevention. Kathy brings the opinions and reactions from the direct patient care experience, and I have the opportunity to use my computer skills and knowledge of infection prevention standards and regulations. Together, we combine our strengths and make a great team. The opportunity to work with a group of nurses from different areas in the hospital has opened my eyes to other projects that were developing at the same time.

I can attest to the fact that strength can be gained for the professional spirit of nursing in every step of the EBP process. The process associated with EBP is a venue to tap into the knowledge we gain as nurses in our everyday experiences and direct the focus to a goal, backed with documentation from reputable literature. Knowledge is strength. If nurses continue to broaden their experiences and knowledge, the professional spirit of nursing will be strengthened.

I am so glad I took the chance and followed through with the experience. I have gained friends in areas of the hospital where I would not have otherwise had the opportunity to work. I have gained knowledge and confidence of the process to support or change a practice with evidence for better patient care. I believe the process has strengthened my skills in areas that support my growth as a nurse. I have also found that I am not alone in my journey; many people in many areas of the hospital are willing to help if asked. My advice to nurses is if you have a gnawing question or concern about patient care, take it to the next level and search for answers. You will gain so much in the process. A passionate journey makes the destination so much richer.

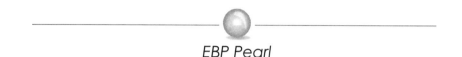

EBP Pearl

With the help of evidence-based mentors, EBP reignites the professional spirit and enthusiasm of clinicians for their roles.

Are You Following the MAP?

–Diane Swintek, BSN, RN, CPAN
Franklin Square Hospital Center
Monkton, Maryland

During the early 1970s when I was in nursing school, evidence-based practice (EBP) was not a requirement for nursing students. Students were expected to conduct a literature search, but it was on a topic selected for us. My inquisitive nature led me to EBP and nursing research decades later in my nursing career. It started with curiosity about my patients who had undergone carotid endarterectomy. At times, these patients had profound bradycardia and/or hypotension, which I closely monitored while they were in my care in the post-anesthesia care unit (PACU). How did I determine that they were hemodynamically stable in the presence of this hypotension and ready to transition to the next level of care? I was utilizing the mean arterial pressure (MAP) to assess for adequate perfusion, but was this supported with science? I performed a literature search in our medical library and quickly realized from the numerous articles generated that a more thorough review of the literature was needed. For me, this EBP project was not only about using the MAP to more efficiently intervene in patient care, but also as a map, as in a chart, to guide me through the entire EBP process: from searching the literature, to critically appraising the evidence, and finally to implementing a practice change in my institution and professional organization.

It was at this time that I had an opportunity to submit an application for the first cohort of evidence-based practice interns in my organization. In January 2008, I was honored and delighted to be selected as one of four EBP interns in our organization. My project was to evaluate the use of MAP in the PACU as a tool to assess hemodynamic stability in patients. My goal was to educate PACU nurses about MAP so that they could better advocate for their patients through earlier hemodynamic intervention to decrease adverse events in the PACU and transition the adult postsurgical patient to the appropriate level of care in a timely fashion.

After I was accepted as an EBP intern, I received guidance from Dr. Carol Esche, CNS in evidence-based practice and research, in formulating a PICO question and identifying and implementing a plan of action. I found the search for evidence utilizing the MAP to determine hemodynamic stability intriguing. Framing the question was difficult, and I went through seven variations, each more discriminating, before reaching my "jumping off" point. It took me a bit of time, weeks in fact, to learn how to read and then critically appraise the literature. The problem I encountered was in searching for evidence in my particular clinical setting: the PACU. Finally, I narrowed the search down to 10 specific articles that included the MAP as a variable used to determine hemodynamic stability. To my dismay, I had to accept that there is no evidence specific to my clinical area of study and that I had to utilize studies evaluating MAP based on research conducted in the intensive care unit (ICU). It was my goal to translate the practice of measuring MAP and intervening in patient care based on these results from the ICU setting to the PACU setting. One particular article by an Australian author addressed critical thinking and decision-making by nurses in the ICU and compared experienced nurses to new nurses. I wrote the author to ask about a possible correlation of that study with the question I was pursuing. I was thrilled when I received a response from this research group in Australia and developed a collegial relationship with them.

Then came the second phase of this project: getting my nurse colleagues to understand the importance of my EBP question and for all of us to have the same basic understanding of the importance of MAP in the PACU setting.

Using some of the articles I had previously identified, I developed and presented an educational program on the significance of the MAP to the PACU nurses. I presented this information to pre- and postanesthesia nurses through a slide presentation and handouts. I explained how I identified the importance of the need to evaluate MAP and presented a review of the literature regarding MAP. In addition, I taught the nursing staff an easy way to determine the MAP using the resources they already had available to them. Finally, I revised the patient care flow sheet to include a column for recording MAP. Initially, this was conducted as a pilot. After everything was tweaked the way it needed to be, I revised our policies to reflect this change in clinical practice. I really felt that this was my opportunity to improve patient care by educating nurses to evaluate the MAP in their patients and to initiate interventions before a crisis. I wanted to do the best job possible. My nurse colleagues initially closely assessed for MAP in their patients and intervened appropriately. However, when I noticed that over time they started to do a perfunctory recording of the MAP, I moved into placing strategic posters in the unit to highlight why careful monitoring of the MAP can improve patient outcome. Just then, I received another note from the Australian author asking about the progress of my project. Her encouragement spurred me on to opening a dialogue within my specialty nursing practice organization, the American Society of PeriAnesthesia Nurses (ASPAN) about utilizing the MAP to determine the stability and readiness of our patients to transition to the next level of care.

I felt it important to disseminate the results of my project. I presented my initial search for evidence as a poster presentation at our state nurses' association conference and did a follow-up poster about the educational design for a national EBP conference sponsored by a university in my area. These two events exposed me to others just like me—the bedside nurse as a nurse investigator. My goal is to write a manuscript based on the outcomes of this project.

This has been a broadening experience for me and has led to my belief that each nurse is capable of contributing to the body of evidence regarding the practice of nursing. I find myself selecting seminar topics that focus on nursing research/EBP so that I can continue to learn how to incorporate this into my nursing practice. EBP is a lot like patient care—it's all about the evidence, and the possibilities are infinite. For me, evaluating MAP in my patients using the EBP process also provided a map to guide me through a complicated but necessary scientific process to assure that I was making a change in practice based on the most current research available. My hope is that EBP will be a map for all nurses to follow as they seek to improve patient care outcomes in all settings.

EBP Pearl

A spirit of inquiry, Step 0 in the EBP process, leads to EBP changes that improve patient care.

Tattoos, Epidurals, and Evidence

–Mark Welliver, DNP, ARNP, CRNA
Associate Professor of Professional Practice,
School of Nurse Anesthesia
Harris College of Nursing and Health Sciences,
Texas Christian University, Fort Worth, Texas

–Dawn Dalpe Welliver, MS, ARNP, CRNA (DNP student)
Staff Nurse Anesthetist and President,
Welliver Anesthesia Corporation, Florida
DNP student, Harris College of Nursing and Health Sciences,
Doctor of Nursing Practice program
Texas Christian University, Fort Worth, Texas

As a certified registered nurse anesthetist (CRNA) on in-house trauma call, I was asked to come to the exceptionally busy obstetrical floor to assist another CRNA in placing epidural catheters in the patients. After placing an epidural catheter without incident, I came to the next patient, Mrs. S, who also requested an epidural catheter for childbirth. After reviewing the chart, performing a history and physical, explaining the risks and benefits, and obtaining informed consent, I prepared the necessary supplies. After positioning the patient, I opened the patient's gown to do a preliminary assessment of the landmarks and site. To my surprise, I observed a large colorful tattoo design in the lumbar region. The tattoo, with multiple swirls and shadings, was truly a work of art, but one that caught me by surprise. Landmark confirmation disclosed the tattoo was in the exact location desired for a lumbar epidural catheter insertion. Because I had not encountered this previously, my immediate question was, "Are there any contraindications to epidural catheter insertion through a tattoo?" Despite remaining current on the literature and questioning several other practitioners, I could find no definitive answers. Assessing my options, I derived the following:

1. Decline the epidural insertion.

2. Proceed with placement through the tattoo.

3. Proceed with placement but avoid piercing the tattoo ink itself.

Using a decision-making process that incorporated a needs assessment, risk-benefit ratio, and informed consent, I proceeded to place the epidural catheter. Rather than directly pierce the tattoo design itself, I placed slight traction on the skin to distract the non-inked skin midline and localized and pierced this ink-free dermis. I placed the epidural catheter without difficulty, tested it, and found it functional. Despite feeling comfortable that this clinical situation was addressed, I felt that the issue was not settled.

Upon returning home the next day, I discussed these events with my spouse, who also is a CRNA and doctor of nursing practice (DNP) student. We proposed four main safety concerns related to placing epidural catheters through low back tattoos:

1. Are there any specific risks associated with tattoo pigments?

2. Does coring of tissues occur with epidural introducer needles?

3. Does tissue transfer occur with introducer needle punctures?

4. Are tattoo pigment components safe in the epidural or intrathecal spaces?

A discussion over coffee moved to the office computer, and we began a Google Scholar search. Initial search terms *tattoo* and *epidural catheter* literally returned thousands of related sources. Reviewing many of these papers and refining our search criteria and database choices, we discovered a paucity of literature that guided or directed practice for our specific concern. Because I had recently finished my DNP studies and my wife was undertaking her DNP studies, we sought to formally explore this clinical concern with the hope of establishing a clearer understanding of the safety or risks involved. Hence, an idea was born: We would perform an evidence-based review with the specific goal of making practice recommendations regarding placement of epidural catheters through low back tattoos.

After forming a team that consisted of ourselves, a nursing faculty instructor and CRNA, and an obstetrical anesthesiologist, we proceeded to systematically review and critically appraise the literature. The key findings were published in the following article:

> Welliver, D., Welliver, M., Carroll, T., & James, P. (2010). Lumbar epidural catheter placement in the presence of low back tattoos: A review of the concerns. *American Association of Nurse Anesthetists Journal*, 78(3), 197–201.

Key findings are as follows:

1. Coring of biological tissues occurs with spinal and epidural needle punctures.

2. Channeling and transfer of bacteria, cells, and potentially pigments can occur with needle punctures of the dermis.

3. Tattoo pigments are natural or synthesized organic and inorganic compounds that may be irritating, allergenic, or carcinogenic.

4. Red pigment is associated with the highest incidence of reactions.

5. The additives in tattoo pigments are not regulated nor fully disclosed to users.

6. Redness, irritation, or infection at a desired epidural site is a contraindication to placement (standard of practice; Welliver, Welliver, Carroll, & James, 2010).

The knowledge of evidence-based clinical assessment, critical thinking, and ultimately application and improvement of clinical practice that the DNP provides has enabled us to explore, evaluate, and contribute to practice improvement. The DNP also has enabled us to educate APRNs, CRNAs, and physician colleagues toward the purpose and benefits of the DNP. Furthermore, communications with several European investigators precipitated by our publication has disclosed additional areas of study regarding this clinical concern. Literature shows tattoo pigments are encapsulated within macrophages as a physiologic response to the foreign material. Do macrophage-encapsulated tattoo pigments isolate the chemicals that might potentially cause harm if tissue coring occurs? Are all tattoo pigments fully encapsulated and isolated from surrounding tissues? Does tissue coring disrupt the encapsulated pigments, exposing them to surrounding tissues? These questions warrant further investigation and might serve to further improve and guide practice. Exploration of these questions is planned. As with all research, more questions are formulated as more knowledge is acquired.

The knowledge and tools obtained through our DNP degree programs enable nurses to better evaluate and guide current clinical practice. This exemplar illustrates a goal of the DNP that strives to improve clinical practice based on collected and critically appraised evidence. We offer clinical guidance where none existed previously and have based these rationales on weighted evidence. The health care system's embrace of evidence-based practice endorses the clinical rationales nurses have used for years when planning patient care. The more structured and systematic approach to this evidence application reinforces that we, as nurses, were on the right track all along.

EBP Pearl

Do not be content when there is no answer to your clinical question; seek out the evidence to answer your question and disseminate it so that others can learn from it.

Who, Me? Tales From an Unexpected Evidence-Based Practice Convert

–Maribeth Gallagher, MS, PMHNP-BC
Dementia Program Director
Hospice of the Valley, Phoenix, Arizona

For years, I acknowledged the importance of evidence-based practice and how it is essential to improve health care. I applauded the endeavors of my nurse colleagues who actively pursued evidence-based efforts, but I never viewed myself as someone suited for participation in the process. As a person who consistently used to shy away or suffer from fits of yawning when I heard discussions of "research findings" or "statistical outcomes," I concluded that EBP was not my "cup of tea." Little did I realize how wrong I was in that assumption. Life is full of wonderful surprises.

In my practice as a psychiatric nurse practitioner specializing in palliative dementia care, I experienced numerous frustrations related to the status quo dementia care that has remained relatively unchanged over the past 30 years. My pursuit of learning about EBP was born far from any natural inclination towards scholarly endeavors, but rather through my deep belief that there must be a better way to do things, coupled with a passion to serve my patients to the best of my ability. I was frustrated with the common practice of relying upon medications to "manage" the behaviors of persons with dementia. I questioned if this practice was truly the only alternative we had to offer such a vulnerable group of elders.

From previous experiences, I'd witnessed people who had done wonderful work trying to change care practices only to have their efforts fail at some point because of a lack of evidence to convince larger audiences and key stakeholders to invest in the practice change. I'd also seen innovative ideas succeed in trial implementations, but fail to be sustained over time. I realized that I needed to explore the full EBP process if I was serious about making a significant and sustainable contribution to dementia care, so I began my journey towards becoming an EBP advanced practice nurse.

By enrolling in the doctor of nursing practice (DNP) program, I learned all the steps of the EBP process through implementation of a small EBP project. I crafted a PICO question to drive my search through the scientific literature for evidence of nonpharmacologic methods to prevent or minimize behaviors in patients with dementia. I became proficient in exploring multiple databases and gathered an impressive array of evidence suggesting effective alternative approaches to dementia care that require little to no medications. Aha! I became even more encouraged when I contacted the authors of the articles I gathered and they offered their support for my EBP endeavors.

I stumbled along the way while evaluating and synthesizing the evidence. It left me feeling frustrated and intellectually clumsy at times, and I reconsidered on more than one occasion whether the EBP process and I were compatible. Numerous unforeseen challenges arose during the actual implementation of my project that tempted me to question my abilities and if the outcome would actually be worth all my efforts. Fortunately, I had a toddler visiting my home, and I realized he never seemed to berate himself or quit trying every time he failed while attempting to learn to walk. I noticed he kept at it, bit by bit, until he succeeded. The toddler became my role model for developing a new attitude towards how to proceed in the EBP process. I silenced my doubts and negative self-talk and simply focused on one step at a time, taking moments to breathe deeply, eat chocolate, and play with my dog. Learning the process did not come easily, but with perseverance and trust in mentors to guide my novice steps, over time I grew an array of skills that ultimately have enhanced my abilities to use my life to make a true difference.

It has been extremely rewarding to see my coauthored publications in professional journals and to hear how they have influenced practice changes around the country. I am energized when I hear about health care professionals experiencing a renewed enthusiasm about the positive impact they can make. Most of all, I can experience no better feeling than when I hear how individual patients with advanced dementia have experienced increased comfort, joy, compassion, and quality of life through methods that I helped disseminate.

One of the most exciting aspects of EBP collaboration is working with global partners who share interests in palliative dementia care. My colleagues and I have disseminated our work throughout the United States, Asia, and parts of Europe and the Middle East. On January 1, 2011, our story appeared on the front page of *The New York Times*. It was entitled "THE VANISHING MIND: Giving Alzheimer's Patients Their Way, Even Chocolate." I was amazed at the outpouring of responses from readers around the world, thousands in the first 24 hours after the story broke. This left me with an indelible lesson—never underestimate the powerful nature of an idea whose time has come. If you feel an idea stirring within you, please listen deeply, because it might be calling you to actualize it into the world. I am humbled when I consider how EBP implementation has used a person like me to influence practice changes that have rippled so far and wide, and I have never experienced such a purposeful and meaningful existence as I do now.

My hopes for you are the same. May your journey into the EBP process lead you to yet-to-be-imagined and deeply fulfilling places.

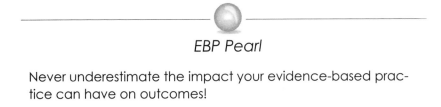

EBP Pearl

Never underestimate the impact your evidence-based practice can have on outcomes!

Innovating Health Care With Evidence-Based Practice

Innovation is an idea that becomes a sustainable reality. Ongoing innovation is the consistent introduction of something radical or new that leads to positive change. Innovation is so needed in the current health care system to enhance the quality of care being delivered across the nation and for the ultimate purpose of improving patient outcomes. In order for clinicians, health care administrators, and policymakers to place their utmost confidence in innovations, they must have a sound evidence base to support them. Further, sustainability of best practice innovations will only occur within cultures that support innovative evidence-based practice.

The stories in this chapter are examples of innovations that have taken place in health care systems across the United States. These stories will appeal to your emotions and move you to think outside of the box to improve care and outcomes for your patients.

The Story of Kim

–Eve Marie Holzemer, DNPc, MSN, RN, ANP
Assistant Professor
Saint Louis University Department of Neurology & Psychiatry, St. Louis, Missouri

Prior to becoming a nurse practitioner, I worked for about 18 years in critical care. While pursuing my advanced degree, I continued to work in this area. I was always one to "push the envelope," and I was always trying to take the team along with me for the ride! One day, we admitted a 24-year-old new mother with a severe stroke. She had given birth about 2 weeks prior to her admission. She had been to her local hospital emergency department with complaints of a severe headache and was sent home with pain medication. She collapsed at home and was flown by helicopter to us in cardiopulmonary collapse. She was what we considered "a real train wreck," on the ventilator, poor oxygenation, on medication to support her BP, and kept paralyzed so that we could maintain her oxygenation. Her condition was so critical that she had multiple specialists attending her. During their rounds, it became apparent that they did not believe she could possibly survive this tremendous complication from a stroke. It was disheartening to see all of the teams making rounds, shaking their heads after examining her, leaving her room, and mumbling that she was probably not going to survive this condition. I was mad as hell. I decided that our nursing team had to act. Several weeks had gone by with no improvement, but only more complications for this young mother. She was so critically ill that we could not leave her room because of the minute-to-minute changes that would occur. We could not get her into the CT or MRI scanner because we could not keep her oxygen level stable.

After much thought, I assembled our nursing team and challenged them to think outside the box. I proposed that we had not done all we could for this young mother and asked them to think of other strategies. I proposed that we have the husband tape record the baby crying and making noises, and we could play that at the head of her bed, which we did. I can still remember walking into this adult unit when my shift would begin, hearing the crying of a baby and remembering that it was only a tape! Interestingly enough, about a week later, things began to stabilize. We continued playing the tapes for another week, and she became even more stable, allowing us to take her for a brain scan and perform a tracheostomy for her long-term ventilatory needs.

Because of her recent progress, paralytic agents were discontinued to see if she would wake up. The real battle began then. We did not have open visiting time (even though the literature supported this), and we certainly did not allow children or babies in the ICU. I was about to start that battle. I rationalized that this was imperative because if this mother survived, we were setting up this family for an attachment disorder because of the lack of bonding between mother and child. I called Kim's husband with my proposal, and he enthusiastically brought the baby to the ICU whenever we summoned him. Many people fought against these concepts, but in the end, whenever this mother opened her eyes, her baby was in the room with her. We would hold the baby over her and tell her, "Your baby is here and needs you to take care of her."

One day I walked into the unit after several days off, and I walked past Kim's room. There she was, wide awake, holding her baby with tears streaming down her face. It was a beautiful sight. We put signs up to keep the medical teams out whenever we had "baby time." We were afraid that if they forgot to wash their hands, she could experience even more complications, and we wanted to prevent any setbacks. To their credit, they respected this time and stayed out of the room whenever the baby was with her mother.

As I consider this patient, a vivid memory occurs. Kim was still on the ventilator, but she was sleeping. Her infant daughter was lying in her lap, also asleep. The baby would rise and fall in timing with the ventilator, the room was dark, and Kim's mother was sleeping peacefully in a chair beside her bed. A frightened medical student was standing outside of the room, trying to grasp the enormity of what he was seeing and wondering why a nurse just told him he could not enter that room. In the end, this patient was with us for 3 months until transferring to rehab, where she recovered for another 3 months. A year later, she came to visit us. Her only disability was weakness in one arm. Her bond with her daughter was strong, and the family survived and thrived. After this, I was able to push for opening visiting hours and including families in the process of critical care. I have always believed that patients are not admitted in isolation, but are part of a system that is imperative to utilize and respect.

EBP Pearl

Your clinical expertise (innovation) combined with scientific knowledge can make the difference between life and death for patients!

Helping Veterans Heal Faster: Innovative "Pet" Therapy

–Darlene Dietrich, MSN, RN, MBA
Nurse Manager Unit 4-West
Veterans Affairs Pittsburgh Healthcare System, Pittsburgh, Pennsylvania

Real animals are not allowed on 4-West, a postsurgery ward in the Veterans Affairs (VA) Pittsburgh Healthcare System. Yet thanks to a unique program called "Operation Walk the Dog," a rotating cast of some 25 dogs—and even a few cats—play a crucial role in patients' recovery. The program, which launched in early 2009 and is the first of its kind in the VA, utilizes a gallery of laminated 8x10 photos of furry friends to get patients moving after surgery. Research shows that there are a lot of benefits to getting up and moving around after an operation.

The whole inspiration behind this program was the common daily activity of walking the dog. Nurses would say to patients, "You have to walk your dog today, so why don't you get up?" Patients can choose to not participate in the program, but those who participate are free to name their adopted dog with the most popular moniker being Butch. These veterans keep the pet's picture in their hospital room throughout their stay. When the veterans take "man's best friend" for a stroll, they often hang the pet's photo from their IV pole or around their neck. The end result is that we always have dogs on the floor! It's a pretty fun—and effective—program.

The purpose of the project was to engage and involve patients in their recovery process. It was heartwarming because patients really enjoyed picking out their "dog" and became attached to her/him as they kept the photo during their stay. The nurses and physical therapists also used the dog pictures as a tool to motivate patients to ambulate. The tactic worked, and patients were seen ambulating more frequently. It was a fun activity to initiate on a postsurgical unit. A side social benefit was the conversation starter the program offered for patients and providers. It was an innovative activity to initiate on a postsurgical unit that demonstrated how nurses can use evidence to change practice in creative and patient-centered ways.

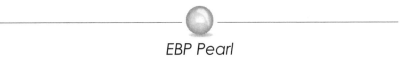

EBP Pearl

EBP innovation encompasses thinking "outside of the box" and comes in many forms to improve patient outcomes!

It's "Mr. R" Again! Improving Perioperative Care of the Patient With Undiagnosed Obstructive Sleep Apnea

–Kathleen Susan Bracy, RN
Staff Nurse
Blessing Hospital, Quincy, Illinois

I literally must have taken care of "Mr. R" a hundred times before. He was in my nursing unit so often that, as soon as I knew it was him, I could predict the course of his stay and his problems.

He came to me for nursing care after his various surgeries and anesthetics. His recovery period was often prolonged. Airway management was often difficult. Pain management was often a nightmare. Anesthetic agents and opioids often impaired his respiratory function. He does not realize it, but he has an increased risk for serious complications. Without proper care, his condition could be life threatening after he left me and went home or to another clinical unit without monitoring.

Often, I knew it was "Mr. R" shortly after he was rolled into my hospital's postanesthesia care unit (PACU) on a stretcher or bed. Sometimes it was difficult for me to recognize him right away when he did not act or look like his characteristic self. This is because "Mr. R" is not always the same patient. He could be male or female, young or old; he could have had a complex 8-hour surgery or an outpatient procedure. You see, "Mr. R" is any patient with undiagnosed obstructive sleep apnea (OSA).

OSA has been around for many years. It is fairly common, but the exact incidence is unknown because people often do not know they have it. And that is exactly what makes it a problem for me and the other direct care nurses like me.

We knew we needed to do something for these patients. How could we make it both easier for the staff and safer for that patient facing surgery and anesthesia? We needed a screening tool to identify patients at risk for OSA and a follow-up plan to care for them.

We used evidence-based practice (EBP) to develop our screening tool. The tool is used either by nurses in our preadmission area when making preoperative calls or by nurses at the surgeon's office. Questions include the following:

- Do you snore?

- Do you ever choke, gasp, or hold your breath when sleeping?

- Do you tire easily during waking hours?

- Do you have high blood pressure?

We also ask height and weight to determine if the body mass index (BMI) is over 35. The "yes" answers are added, with 3 indicating moderate risk and 4 or more positive answers indicating high risk of OSA.

We then developed the OSA Respiratory Precaution Orders Set in conjunction with the anesthesiologist. Now, when "Mr. R" comes into the PACU, he has already been identified as a moderate or high risk for OSA. I know right away that this patient has specific needs. I use the orders to guide my care regarding length of observation, respiratory treatments, and postoperative monitoring. We also use end tidal CO_2 monitoring on these patients. CO_2 monitoring is also based on EBP, identifying respiratory depression more effectively and earlier than pulse oximetry alone. We give the patient an education brochure to provide teaching about OSA and encourage the patient to follow up with their primary care physician for possible treatment. I arrange admission or prolonged recovery if the patient requires it.

Much education was required for the many disciplines involved to get these changes going and implement them successfully. Any new change is not easy at first. We all know resistance often exists, like the frequently heard complaints, "Another new project?" or "Just more work for me to do." I have worked as a direct care registered nurse in the PACU for nearly 30 years. I have heard the familiar "that's how we always do it here" many times and have said it myself. I admit that I used to groan and roll my eyes when

I heard about EBP. I didn't even know what it involved. But now, with increased understanding and after seeing EBP in action in other nursing units during our hospital's recent Magnet Journey, I truly find nursing more exciting than ever. We as staff nurses can use EBP to change care from "what we have done because we have always done it that way" to "what we currently do because it is better." We can make improvements in nursing care and, more importantly, patient outcomes. The changes we made in our initiative for OSA have been huge. We will continue to review new EBP literature as it becomes available.

I continue to care for "Mr. R" many times. Since our initiative, we have found that 10% of our patients are at high risk and 30% are at moderate risk for OSA. That makes for a frequent repeat customer. The next time "Mr. R" comes into PACU, I know he will have care that is improved from how it was "always done."

Now, I have a consistent plan of care for "Mr. R." I will be ready in PACU because I know ahead of time when he is coming. "Mr. R" will get the same quality of care regardless of which nurse or which anesthesiologist cares for him. He will be monitored so any complications can be treated quickly and resolved. I know he will get continued monitoring as needed when he leaves me and I feel good because his safety is so important to me. I feel that patient education could be one of the best outcomes. Maybe "Mr. R" will learn about OSA, talk to his physician, and get the treatment he needs to avoid lifelong health problems from OSA.

These changes based on EBP will help him *and* me a lot.

EBP Pearl

EBP reduces the variation in practice and assures that all patients receive the highest quality of care and attain the best outcomes.

DNP and EBP: Here Comes the Judge

–Madelaine Binner, DNP, MBA, CRNP-BC
Medical Oncology Nurse Practitioner, Sidney Kimmel Comprehensive Cancer Center
Johns Hopkins Bayview Medical Center, Pasadena, Maryland

I have a 77-year-old female patient who has metastatic carcinoid of the small bowel. She has had surgery and chemoembolization of hepatic lesions and continued with carcinoid syndrome symptoms (lots of diarrhea). She had failed to control her diarrhea on Lomotil and Imodium (15 stools/day) and was hospitalized twice for dehydration and electrolyte imbalance. She had been receiving octreotide injections monthly. Tincture of opium was then added with good effect during her last hospitalization.

Subsequently, Medicare Part D declined to pay for her prescription for tincture of opium as it has never been formally FDA approved; it existed and was used for diarrhea control for 2500 years, pre-FDA existence. The basis of the denial was that the insurer claimed they did not have to provide drug coverage for non-formulary and/or non-FDA approved medications (they provided the documentation to support their denial).

I appealed to Medicare on the patient's behalf and was twice denied. So I then appealed to the court for a hearing by a Medicare Administrative Law Judge. At first, the thought of presenting my argument to a judge was very intimidating. I decided my best argument was to produce the evidence. As a new doctor of nursing practice (DNP) graduate, I used my newly developed skills to search databases for evidence supporting my position. My letters and documentation of the evidence were submitted as Exhibits 1 and 2 for the hearing proceedings.

In the Judge's analysis, it was noted that:

> *The record clearly establishes that tincture of opium was commercially used or sold in the United States before the date of the enactment of the Drug Amendments of 1962 and that it has not been the subject of a final determination by the Secretary that it is a 'new drug'.... Tincture of opium has been used for centuries, and its most recent use is for the control of fulminant diarrhea. Dr. Binner's report establishes that she prescribed tincture of opium to control intractable diarrhea resulting from*

carinoid tumors…. It is not the subject of a final determination by the Secretary that it is a 'new drug' or an action brought by the Secretary under section 301, 302(a), or 304(a) of such Act to enforce section 502(f) or 505(a) of such act. Therefore, tincture of opium is a covered outpatient drug as defined by the statute…. Dr. Binner's conclusions (Exhibit 2/page 21), which are unrebutted, established that tincture of opium is effective and that other drugs on any tier of the Plan's formulary would not be as effective for the Beneficiary as tincture of opium would be. Only tincture of opium has provided any relief (Exhibit 2/page 21). In Dr. Binner's opinion, other formulary drugs such as codeine would have adverse effects for the Beneficiary.

Thus, the record as a whole shows that the prescription drug alternatives listed on the formulary or required to be used in accordance with step therapy requirements have been ineffective in the treatment of the enrollee's disease or medical condition or, based on both sound clinical evidence and medical and scientific evidence and the known relevant physical and mental characteristics of the enrollee and known characteristics of the drug regimen, is likely to be ineffective or adversely affect the drug's effectiveness or patient compliance.

Dr. Binner's report (Exhibit 2/page 21) proves that Lomotil was ineffective and that based on both sound clinical evidence and medical and scientific evidence and the known relevant physical and mental characteristics of the enrollee and known characteristics of the drug regimen, is likely to be ineffective or adversely affect the drug's effectiveness or patient compliance.

For all these reasons, a preponderance of the credible evidence shows that an exception to the formulary is warranted.

The Plan is required to pay for the Appellant's tincture of opium.

An exception to the non-formulary status of tincture of opium is granted, effective immediately.

The Plan is DIRECTED to act in accordance with this order.

I added excerpts of the actual record so that readers can appreciate the complexities of the judicial process. I did not always clearly comprehend all the "legalese," but clearly understood the decision of "Favorable" on behalf of my patient. In the judge's decision, he noted that Dr. Binner provided sufficient evidence that, although tincture of opium was never officially FDA approved and non-formulary, based on Dr. Binner's documentation and submitted evidence, he overturned the denials and now Medicare Part D insurer will have to cover the drug. This translates to a $500/month cost savings for my patient. My patient almost cried when she heard the decision. I wanted to frame the decision letter from the court!

I truly believe that the DNP gave me the skills, the credibility, and the confidence to take on this challenge. Also, it felt really good to have a judge refer to me as Dr. Binner, the patient's provider!

EBP Pearl

Decisions are made and cases are won with solid data; learn to present your arguments for changing practice with solid evidence.

Improving Transplant Patient Education Through Evidence-Based Practice

–Rebecca Brown, BSN, RN, CCTC
Transplant Coordinator
Pinnacle Health System, Harrisburg, Pennsylvania

When patients are faced with the prospect of kidney transplantation to treat their end-stage renal disease (ESRD), they are often completely overwhelmed. Some patients have months or even years to learn about the process, whereas others are referred for transplant evaluation after only one visit with their nephrologist.

As required by the Centers for Medicare & Medicaid Services (CMS), transplant centers must fully inform potential transplant candidates of the risks and benefits of transplantation at the time of initial evaluation. Education of the potential candidate must also include alternative treatments for ESRD and current Scientific Registry of Transplant Recipient (SRTR) graft survival and patient survival statistics. This education includes the candidate evaluation process, the roles of each member of the transplant team, the surgical procedure, immediate and long-term postop care, the necessity of lifelong immunosuppressive medications and their potential side effects, the routine lifelong physician and laboratory visits, the monitoring of vital signs for signs of rejection, and dietary guidelines. Candidates must understand that multifaceted financial issues surround transplantation, including insurance and prescription coverage for immunosuppressive medications and the role that Medicare plays in the ESRD diagnosis. The patient's right to informed consent is strictly followed, affirming that the candidate understands the entire transplant process. In fact, two signed consents are required that verify the candidate's understanding of the entire transplant process: the first at the time of initial evaluation and the second at the time of transplant listing.

Obviously, patients and their family members have a lot of information to absorb and to retain. Prior to implementation of our evidence-based protocol (EBP), the candidate's evaluation process consisted of educational information and a complex patient review that included introduction to the transplant surgeon, a psychosocial evaluation by the social worker, a review of systems by the transplant coordinator, a review of the patient's insurance and prescription plan by the financial counselor, and finally laboratory testing, which includes the drawing of about 23 tubes of blood at the patient's first appointment! This was commonly known as "clinic day" and, in all honesty, it was not only exhausting to the patients, but to the transplant coordinators, too.

The logistics of the clinic were:

1. Clinic began at 7:45 A.M. and usually did not conclude until 1:30 or 2:00 P.M.

2. Four patients with their family members were seen at each session.

3. We used a video (which had become outdated) and lecture format to educate patients.

4. We held clinic twice a week, every week, for 9 years.

This was our routine, and we trudged through it week after week. The coordinators recognized that the patients got fatigued early on in the process, and by the end of the 6-hour appointment, they were not actively participating any more. Candidates and family members did not remember much of the information that was presented, even though substantial printed material was also provided.

Teaching the same information to small groups of patients every week had become more of a chore than a challenge to all the coordinators. We were spending 12 hours, or 30% of our work week, providing formal patient education, and we believed that we were not providing effective education—sometimes patients even fell asleep during our education process! When patients cancelled at the last minute or did not show up for an appointment, we were providing all this information to only one or two patients. If we had very talkative patients, we had to rush through some aspects of the education.

Confounding the clinic process was the reliance on county transportation for some of our patients. Because the appointments began so early and continued into the afternoon, some of the county transportation buses would not assist patients with transportation to these appointments. Our geographical service area is fairly large; therefore, it became a problem to get patients to and from this 6-hour appointment.

It was my goal to develop an EBP that would improve our patient education process. I wanted patients to retain more of the information that they received, and I wanted to do this in a more efficient manner for the nurses, too.

I am currently attending graduate school and was dreading having to take another nursing research class last summer—after all, because I am a perpetual student who started her nursing career in an ADN program, moved to a BSN program, and am now back in school again pursuing my MSN, I have had my fair share of nursing research classes! Taking an optimistic approach, I decided to use my research project to improve my nursing practice. After an extensive review of both transplantation literature and adult education concepts, I was able to develop an EBP that could be put into practice fairly easily at our center. I was very fortunate to have the support of all my colleagues and my director to initiate this much-needed change.

Our center now provides group patient education three times per month. The education class starts at 9:00 A.M., and we strongly encourage each potential recipient to bring their family members or other support people and any potential living kidney donors to this appointment. I developed a PowerPoint presentation for this educational class, and we stopped using our outdated videos. This group education class is about 90 minutes in length, and it is a requirement that patients attend prior to beginning their evaluation.

The presentation has improved our practice in many ways—because this appointment has been shortened, retention of information has improved. We have had many patients comment on the content of the presentation and how much they learned at the session. Several patients have commented that they have received more information about the transplant process during this session than they have at other centers where they have been evaluated. In addition, patients have commented about the cartoons and pictures that are used, which we believe validates retention of the information.

The PowerPoint also has ensured consistency of information presented by the different coordinators. Three coordinators present this information. This format ensures that we all discuss the same information at each session—even when we are sidetracked by patient questions. The other benefit to this format is that patients bring their family members to the session, and the entire family learns about the process. Every nurse knows that chronic illness never affects only the person with the disease, but their entire support system. Our center places a very strong emphasis on providing education to the entire family to improve post-transplant outcomes and patient satisfaction.

The next step in our process is the patient evaluation. This is scheduled after the education class, usually within one or two weeks. The evaluation process has not changed much. The patients still meet with the coordinator, surgeon, financial counselor, and social worker on this day, but the appointment is now shortened to 3 hours or less, and it starts at 10:00 A.M.—no more complaints about rush hour traffic in the capitol of Pennsylvania! Patients arrive refreshed to the appointment, and it is evident that they have retained information from the education class because they usually bring necessary information that was discussed at the education session.

The goal for this project was to increase retention of transplant education and to improve patient satisfaction. We have achieved that goal and discovered benefits for the coordinators, too! Changing our process has allowed us more time to provide individualized care for our patients. It also has improved our attitudes. We enjoy providing this patient education—it is a more interactive process as patients are given ample time for questions and answers. We can stress the importance of bringing necessary medical records to the evaluation appointment, which cuts down on the amount of time that we are spending trying to retrieve records, and we don't have many patients sleeping through the education anymore.

The impetus for this EBP was an assignment for my nursing research class; however, being able to put this into practice was the most rewarding element of the assignment. I was able to recognize a problem, review available evidence on the subject, and improve patient outcomes and staff satisfaction. My professor's challenge to develop a project that would be practical was all I needed to change a process that was outdated. I know that I will continue to utilize and develop evidence-based protocols in my practice.

EBP Pearl

Furthering your education can enhance your EBP skills *and* benefit your patients and the staff with whom you work.

From Prison Research to Evidence-Based Reentry Support Program for Women and Children

–Mary W. Byrne, PhD, MPH, NP, FAAN
Stone Foundation and Elise Fish Professor of Health Care for the Underserved
Columbia University School of Nursing, New York, New York

I first went to prison in the late 1990s. I was not convicted of a crime nor was I am employee of the Department of Corrections. I am among the few research scientists given Institutional Review Board approvals and state corrections department entree to conduct research with incarcerated women over several years. My voluntary time in prison comprised regularly scheduled study visits for intervention and data collection as principal investigator on a study funded by the National Institute of Nursing Research entitled

"Maternal and Child Outcomes of a Prison Nursery." When the study was completed, a group of civilian employees and volunteers within the prison adopted part of the protocol and found resources to make that a sustainable addition to the prison services offered to child-rearing women who had completed their sentences and were being released.

As a nurse scientist focused on interventional support for stressed parents of infants and toddlers in community settings, I found the opportunity to study outcomes of women and children inside a prison nursery a welcome and daunting challenge. The relatively rapid translation of empirical data into one viable and continuing evidence-based program adopted by the prison system itself was an unanticipated benefit of this experience. This proximate application of research evidence to innovative practice has been inspiring and professionally satisfying. This paper traces the journey from funded research project to the adopted new evidence-based program. It is a journey across disciplines, social systems, and people's intersecting lives.

A prison nursery provides coresidence inside a correctional facility for a pregnant woman convicted of a felony crime and her infant for whom she remains the primary caregiver. These arrangements exist globally, but are relatively uncommon in the United States. In 2010, seven states (Indiana, Illinois, Nebraska, New York, Ohio, South Dakota, and Washington) had prison nursery programs. They offer coresidence for incarcerated mothers and their infants for anywhere from 30 days through 30 months. More typically, newborns are separated from their incarcerated mothers within 24 to 48 hours after birth and placed in the custody of family members or into the foster care system. The majority of mothers do not receive visits from their children throughout their incarcerations, and telephone calls are restricted and expensive. The few prison-based coresidence programs have had brief and fragmented histories and limited resources to meet new mothers' health needs. No rigorous evaluations have been undertaken; even demographic reports are sparse. New York State supports arguably the oldest of the nation's prison nursery programs, which was established in a girls' reformatory in 1901 and has continued in what is now the state's maximum security prison for women and in an adjacent medium security women's prison. These were the settings for the study.

Prison-based research has had a tainted history in the United States and was briefly halted completely in the early 1970s following public disclosure that diseases were deliberately induced in prisoners. Formation of the National Commission for the Protection of Human Subjects of Biomedical and Behavioral Research resulted in passage of the National Research Act in 1974 to protect human subjects. Protections were added later specific to pregnant women, prisoners, and finally children. At the present time, the Code of Federal Regulations, Title 45, Part 46 (45 CFR 46) regulates human subject participation in all federally funded studies and commercially sponsored pharmaceutical trials.

To conduct the research study described, I met all 45 CFR 46 requirements, received university institutional review board (IRB) full review and approval, applied successfully to the research division of the corrections system, and exercised the option to apply for a federal Certificate of Confidentiality, which provides the researcher with the ability to resist most legal demands for disclosure of subject information. Additional measures were taken to build the trust needed for a long-term collaboration. Though not required, I sought frequent meetings with all levels of administrative, civilian, and inmate groups, especially when personnel changes were made or regulations altered. The first in a series of studies was an ethnography of mothering in a prison nursery. This established a foundation of researcher and participant as coinvestigators. The sharing philosophy underlying ethnographic methods was maintained throughout the subsequent quantitative cross-sectional and longitudinal studies.

The specific aims of the first longitudinal research study were to (1) compare the impact of nursing interventions on parent-child interaction, parenting competency, and child development; (2) measure attachment achieved by infants in the prison nursery and maintained during the transition to community; and (3) identify short-term criminal recidivism of the prison nursery mothers. Rolling recruitment resulted in a cohort of 100 mother-infant dyads who provided written informed consent (with only one eligible women refusing). Using several standard questionnaires, the Adult Attachment Interview and the Bayley Scales of Infant Development, data were collected throughout the prison nursery coresidency and during the first year in which the infant reentered the free community. Participants received weekly nurse practitioner visits inside prison followed by biweekly telephone and written information and support during the first reentry year. Parent-child interaction and parenting competency saw gains, and all infants met developmental milestones. Although the majority of mothers' internal representation of their own attachment was markedly insecure, women raised infants with measurable secure attachment at rates comparable to healthy community families. During the reentry year, we collected quantitative and qualitative data on the cumulative psycho-social risks mothers and toddlers faced, which threatened the gains made. First reentry year, return-to-prison rates were far lower than rates reported for similar women separated from their children by incarceration.

During the years in which the research was conducted, prison staff became interested in the intervention protocols we were testing. Though all prison nursery programs are assumed to be interventions that improve mothering, achieve attachment, optimize development, and clinch reentry success, only recidivism outcomes had been established with more than anecdotal data. In addition, during the study years, we were testing a structured intervention that provided more than the prison nursery program alone. Nurse visits were provided tailored to individual parenting concerns and to provide information and support on a one-to-one basis. This continued after release through focused telephone conversations and a series of one-page written and pictorial handouts geared to the particular needs of raising infants and toddlers following maternal history of criminal justice involvement. This process resonated with the civilian staff who had worked with the mothers in the prison nursery and who long entertained the need for an ongoing outreach program for newly released mothers. This need was underscored by the unsolicited phone calls staff received from mothers arriving in the community and beset with overwhelming needs for housing, employment, child care, and health care in the face of scarce educational and financial capital.

While our research was in progress, staff asked us to meet with them and describe how we maintained contact with research participants and how they responded. They were impressed with our retention rates approaching 80% for the entire first reentry year. We shared our protocols for identifying release addresses and keeping up with the constantly changing telephone numbers. We all agreed on the need to establish trust, ensure privacy, and offer a program that could be identified as separate from but compatible with the parole offices that directed these women's lives during early reentry. We mutually agreed to share our methodology without identifying details about any particular participants or overreaching the boundaries of confidentiality. Staff maintained their interest in establishing a sustainable program of telephone outreach and support for newly released mothers. Without the resources of research funding and within the constraints of corrections budgeting, this seemed like an illusive goal.

Nevertheless, the staff had several assets on which to capitalize. They established helping relationships while women were on the prison nursery units so they would not be "cold-calling." They had affiliations to facilitate referrals. Another asset was the staff themselves, all educated in human service professions and with experience in criminal justice settings. Added to this was the *sine qua non* quality of knowing how to convey respect and advice to highly stressed individuals, a skill that is learned but not easily taught, a compelling quality of personal effectiveness that was particularly intuitive in the person who hoped to direct the new program.

Shortly after our first study ended, we learned that staff had achieved their first goal. They reviewed their pilot program with us. They received departmental permission to continue and identified budget lines. The program is approaching its third year, and staff are identifying positive outcomes in terms of contacts, referrals, and recidivism. This rapid translation of empirical data to an evidence-based program is the more admirable because it occurred in a resource-sparse and highly controlled setting. Political and economic pressures to reduce recidivism enhanced the timing for support of a reentry program. The ongoing formal and informal communication triggered by the presence of a research study and continued among committed professionals with shared interests in a needy population were the driving force.

EBP Pearl

Findings from research must be rapidly translated into clinical practice to improve care and patient outcomes as well as to reduce the 17-year research-practice time gap.

Code White: A Response to Patients With Massive Hemorrhage

–Martha Clark, BS, RN
Nurse Manager, Surgical Unit
Shore Health System, Easton, Maryland

–Amalia Punzo, MD
Medical Director, Quality Improvement and Patient Safety
Shore Health System, Easton, Maryland

Our hospital system is located on the Eastern Shore of Maryland and is considered a rural community hospital system. We are two hospitals that are part of the larger University of Maryland health care system. We strive to uphold our mission and strategic principle, "Exceptional Care Everyday." We are one of a select few rural hospitals in the country to have achieved Magnet status (October, 2009). We are no strangers to clinical innovation and exemplar professional practice. We also take great pride in investigating our near misses (good catches) and adverse events with the intent of improving our processes and clinical practice. The following is a story of how an event in our birthing center prompted an innovative system-wide initiative to hasten and streamline the rapid response of people, resources, and blood products to the bedside of a patient experiencing a massive hemorrhage.

A little over a year ago, our birthing center experienced a case of profound postpartum hemorrhage and disseminated intravascular coagulation (DIC). Root cause analysis (RCA) of this event revealed that we should develop a more rapid and coordinated interdepartmental response for patients with bleeding emergencies. It also was clear that physicians did not have a consistent evidence-based approach to ordering blood products in proper ratios. As a result of this RCA, the hospital quality team launched a system-wide multidisciplinary task force to streamline our processes and review evidence-based practices in response to a hemorrhagic emergency. We also spoke with numerous hospitals regarding how they handled urgent hemorrhagic crises. The group met monthly and ultimately developed a policy with computerized and paper-based order sets and subsequent system-wide education for what was referred to as a *Code White*.

The group also investigated what resources were needed to more rapidly transfuse blood into these critically ill patients. Subsequently, we ordered two additional rapid blood transfusers, one for each of our hospital campuses. The patient educator for the birthing center developed the education and training plan for nursing. Staff received intensive education on how to use this new equipment and about the new Code White initiative. These types of bleeding emergencies are actually extremely rare at our hospitals and, therefore, we needed to make sure our nurses were periodically inserviced on the use of the rapid transfusers and how to initiate a Code White. The Code White task force was in the process of conducting drills on this new system initiative when my story begins.

I am the nurse manager of the surgical unit. I am also the manager representative of our Nursing Shared Leadership (Shared Governance) Global Team. This team comprises staff nurses from each of our nursing units. At one of the recent Global Team meetings, the birthing center nurse educator presented the new Code White policy and stressed how important this new policy was for the critical care areas, OB, and the EDs. I leaned over to my unit representative and said, "This kind of thing will never happen to us." Our patients typically come out of surgery with their wounds sutured and cauterized!

And so the story goes, I was out walking one very early bright spring morning with my friend and colleague from the hospital blood bank. She was updating me on the progress she was making with her staff regarding their Code White education. She had developed an algorithm for the blood bank staff to use for the thawing, preparation, and release of the necessary blood products. Around the same time frame, the medical director of quality improvement for the system also happened to be updating me regarding the upcoming Code White drills that were being planned in the EDs and birthing center. This is where the story takes a drastic turn.

One afternoon in the fall of 2009, our surgical unit had just accepted transfer of a post-thyroidectomy patient from the PACU. The patient was being wheeled past me as I made my way back to my office. The surgical unit nurse and the PACU nurse were in the process of transferring the patient onto her bed, when all of a sudden I heard staff calling for help and arrived to see bright red blood rapidly escaping from the patient's neck wound. Our unit has never had such an event happen during my tenure as nurse manager. We had not even been formally educated on Code White yet because the hospitals were still in the process of conducting drills. The policy had not even yet been posted. So when I assessed the severity of what was taking place before our eyes, I quickly recalled what I did know about the Code White initiative and asked the unit secretary to call the switchboard operator to page a Code White overhead. It was about 4:00 P.M., and I counted on the blood bank knowing what to do. I knew the staff had been prepared for this rare and serious crisis. Luckily, two of our surgeons were still available in the building. I was certainly grateful for the Code White team that promptly responded. Everyone who was needed showed up within minutes and brought their tools and expertise to the bedside.

The rapid transfuser was transported to the bedside; the blood bank staff hand-delivered the first few units of O negative blood and release forms; a surgeon appeared; and the PACU manager responded and readied the OR and PACU for this patient. Most people, I was later told, thought this was a surprise drill! The patient was transported back to the OR and was in surgery within 10 short minutes. She received four units of blood in a record amount of time via the rapid transfuser. The surgeon continues to comment that she has never witnessed such a prompt response to a hemorrhage. She called the chief medical officer to credit the team and our unit. To make a long but wonderful story short, this patient survived and did well returning home.

EBP Pearl

The use of available evidence combined with teamwork, innovation, and a dedication to excellence improves care and saves patients' lives.

Oh . . . For the Love of Mom and Dad

–Amy Sebastian-Deutsch, DNP, RN, CNS, AOCNS
System Cancer Services
Memorial Hermann Healthcare System, Houston, Texas

In July 2004, I was scheduled for a total proctocolectomy with J-pouch. Mom and Dad decided to drive from Pittsburgh to Houston to stay with my son and to help provide my postoperative (postop) care. During the prior 3 months, Mom had not been feeling well. She had experienced vague, intermittent gastrointestinal (GI) symptoms. Her family doctor prescribed the standard medications for symptomatic relief and ordered a pelvic ultrasound, which he indicated was normal. Later on, we would find out the written report was abnormal and included a suggestion for further follow-up because ascites was noted.

Concerned, I examined Mom's abdomen. During the process, she gasped in pain. I suggested she see my GI doctor and scheduled an appointment. While I was hospitalized, she saw the doctor and had a computerized axial tomography (CT) scan. Six days postop, I was discharged home. The GI doctor called me and stated, "I have bad news about your Mom. This needs to be a conference call. Make sure your Dad is with her." She proceeded to indicate Mom's CT scan showed some type of cancer, probably ovarian. She also stated the CT showed ascites and fluid in her lung. We were devastated with the news . . . *unbelievable* . . . Mom, Granny, Louie (individual names for the matriarch of our family) had CANCER.

During my immediate recovery from major surgery and while trying to absorb the fact I now had an ileostomy, I tried to coordinate Mom's initial care. A pulmonologist performed a thoracentesis that resulted in 1800 cc of fluid with positive cytology, which was consistent with primary peritoneal cancer. We were in shock, and emotions ran high. Yet the old nursing "take charge" attitude kicked in, and I managed to deal with insurance companies, change my ileostomy bag, make doctor appointments for Mom, and accompany her to her oncology and pulmonology visits—all while holding a pillow to my abdomen and slurping on red Gatorade. I was constantly bordering on dehydration with tears always a blink away.

The oncologist indicated Mom would need chemotherapy. All doctors stated it was not safe for her to drive back to Pittsburgh with Dad, but she could fly home if someone accompanied her on a direct flight. My sister arrived to escort Mom. They returned to Pittsburgh where Mom received care by a local oncologist. In September 2004, she began chemotherapy treatments.

She and Dad received verbal instruction about chemotherapy from the nurses, but it was far too much to remember for a 75-year-old, newly diagnosed cancer patient and her 76-year-old husband; both still in shock from the recent diagnosis. During our phone conversations, Mom and Dad verbalized they were anxious about the possible chemotherapy side effects. They had heard stories about chemotherapy from friends and family members. As I talked with them on the telephone and discussed side effects that were occurring, it was apparent that Mom and Dad had not retained much of the information provided by the nurses.

Mom's initial treatment was with six cycles of paclitaxel/carboplatin (TC) and remission lasted 18 months. She was retreated with TC with 9 more months of remission. After relapse, she received several other regimens, which included doxorubicin liposomal, gemcitabine/carboplatin, a hormonal agent, and oral etoposide. With each new regimen came a new set of instructions, and each time, my parents had difficulty remembering what they were told. I thought, with all the pharmaceutical companies in existence, surely there would be a resource available that actually presented this information in a nonthreatening manner.

In 2007, I enrolled in the DNP program at Rocky Mountain University of Health Professions in Provo, Utah. The program focused on the implementation of evidence-based practice (EBP) and required a capstone project. Having finished my master's degree in 1989, EBP was a new concept for me. From my viewpoint, it legitimized nursing. My clinical mentor and I met to discuss possible ideas for a capstone project.

I had just spent 25 years working in oncology and recognized the vital importance of patient teaching. I knew firsthand how difficult it was for my parents to remember what the nurses had taught them pertaining to chemotherapy and how anxious they had been about the treatments. In my heart, I knew quality patient teaching was pivotal. My parents were both educators and had impressed upon my sisters and I the importance of education. This served as the impetus for my EBP project. I went to the literature with the following burning clinical question. "In newly diagnosed cancer patients, how does a chemotherapy patient teaching DVD compared to oral patient teaching by the nurses affect levels of anxiety and depression?"

I believed toxicity profiles could be improved with proper patient teaching. I searched the evidence to determine how using a chemotherapy patient teaching DVD has affected both anxiety and depression. Given our "techno-savvy" culture, I was shocked to find no current chemotherapy video or DVD on the market. I found radiation therapy DVDs, but the most recent chemotherapy video was 9 years old, and it was from Canada. Through my evidence review, I found that education had been shown to decrease anxiety levels as well as increase knowledge. Furthermore, the evidence indicated a majority of cancer patients want to receive education about their treatment. Because at the time I could not find any specific evidence pertaining to the impact of using a DVD for chemotherapy education, my capstone project became a study to answer the research question, "What is the effect of a chemotherapy patient teaching DVD on anxiety and depression in newly diagnosed cancer patients?"

As I continued my planning for my capstone project, I knew, after additional evidence review, that I would use the Hospital Anxiety and Depression Scale (HADS) to measure levels of anxiety and depression pretreatment and posttreatment to evaluate the use of the teaching DVD. There was just one catch. I would need to produce the teaching DVD, and I had absolutely no experience in movie production. Furthermore, I had no idea what it would actually cost to produce a DVD. Little did I know, I was about to learn about barriers to EBP. Even better, I learned how to knock them down!

Starting in January 2008, I interviewed four production companies and was quoted from $10,000 to $48,000 for the project. I had no budgeted money and had to apply for $28,000 in funding to cover the cost of the project—another new experience. I learned if I asked for research funds, the answer was usually no. I discovered that if I requested small amounts of money ($500–$4000) for the development of a chemotherapy patient teaching DVD, the answers were generally yes. Using this knowledge, I obtained sufficient funds to cover production costs.

During this time, I wrote the script and recruited all participants, which included physicians, nurses, a dietitian, a chaplain, a pharmacist, cancer survivors, and a news anchor who would narrate the DVD. I scouted for filming locations and obtained permissions to film and to use Jim Brickman's piano music on the DVD. Filming commenced in August and the days were long and tedious—typically starting at 0600 and ending at 1800. Equipment was set up and taken down multiple times each day with temperatures soaring into the 90s. We even waited for clouds to pass so lighting would be appropriate. It was unbelievable what went into making a quality movie. Though I wanted to stop many times, the excitement of the cancer survivors who participated in the project spurred me on.

And then, it was time to edit 24 hours of film down to 27 minutes, a task I thought impossible, especially when in the middle of September, Hurricane Ike swept through Houston, destroying the production studio. In spite of a hurricane, we finished the DVD, and it premiered late in November 2008. I sent a copy of the DVD to my parents for their input because I knew they would be honest critics. Mom's comment said it all. "Where was this when I was going through chemo? It would have been helpful."

Patients were enrolled into my study after IRB approval. Anxiety scores (as measured by the HADS tool) decreased significantly from pre- to post-viewing of the DVD. Study results confirmed the effectiveness of the DVD as it related to anxiety levels. However, depression scores did not change significantly. To date, 300 copies have been distributed for patient teaching: across our hospital system, in doctors' offices across Houston, coast-to-coast across the United States, and in Pakistan. The DVD has been incorporated into our hospital system chemotherapy patient teaching policy and procedure and is also shown at the beginning of each chemotherapy course for nurses. When finished, I declared I would never produce a DVD again. Well, watch out what you say—a Spanish version has been filmed and has now been released.

Were it not for the patience and perseverance exhibited by Mom and Dad over the years, and demonstrated so recently in their cancer journey, this DVD might have never come to fruition. Oh, for the love of Mom and Dad, who have traveled the chemotherapy road together.

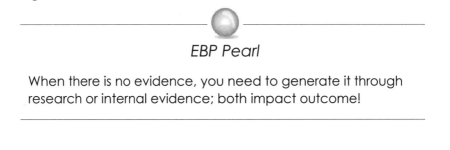

EBP Pearl

When there is no evidence, you need to generate it through research or internal evidence; both impact outcome!

Mother and Baby Survive Cardiac Arrest Due to Research Study

–Lisa A. Gay, MSN, BSN, RN,
Brown Mackie College Nursing Faculty
La Paz, Indiana

On one Friday the 13th, I learned the importance of evidence-based practice. My pregnant 32-year-old daughter and her husband were attending "movie night" at their church when she suffered a full arrest. She had no cardiac history and had just been to her prenatal check-up the week before. I had been an OB nurse for several years, and I had not detected any problems.

Thankfully, some people at the gathering were trained in CPR. She was taken to one of the few hospitals in the United States that was participating in a research study that used hypothermia protocols on specific full arrest codes. The premise is that reduction of body temperature reduces the flow of toxins to the brain, thereby conserving neurological function. But problems arose when the hospital personnel realized she was pregnant because this procedure had never been trialed on a pregnant client. Because she was not quite 20 weeks in gestation, it was decided the baby was not viable without the mother, so a very brave emergency room physician opted to include her in the study.

Lowering her body temperature worked, and she survived the first 48 hours. Her arrhythmia continued to be a problem and on her second day on life support, her cardiologists told us she needed to have a defibrillator/pacemaker implanted or she would not survive. But she had aspirated and now had pneumonia with the accompanying fever; thus, she was not a surgical candidate. We prepared for her to die.

One nurse caring for her kept muttering that he had read something in one of the nursing journals about an external defibrillator vest that he thought could buy her time until her fever broke. He spent the next few hours scouring the Internet to get information on the new equipment. At 3:00 A.M., he exclaimed, "I found it!" and without any hesitation, he phoned the cardiologist and awoke him to ask for permission to get the new equipment sent into the hospital. Every nurse knows how daunting it must be to wake a doctor in the wee hours of the morning, much less to ask about obtaining an experimental piece of equipment! The doctor ordered the vest. By dawn a company representative had flown in from out of state, and the cardiologist and I were meeting with him to get our training on the vest that could potentially save her life. I remember being scared about getting the vest up and working in time. But by the time we had completed the training, her fever had broken and she was whisked off to surgery for her new implanted cardio-defibrillator. Fortunately, we didn't need the vest after all, but we were very glad the option had been there. Without the nurse using his evidence-based practice skills, we would never have known about the new equipment and she might have died. We will be forever grateful to his dedication to the profession and to his patients.

I worried about our grandbaby and how much damage we had caused him. He had been oxygen deprived and defibrillated in excess of 20 times. His mother had been without a spontaneous heartbeat for more than 45 minutes. He had been given cardiac medications and chilled to the point you could see him shivering on the ultrasound. His unconscious mother was on life support for more than a week. On a warm day in July, our new grandson entered this world. He is perfect in every way! We nicknamed him Zap because he had been defibrillated so many times. He earned his name, because he is one busy guy!

Our daughter continues to improve. At one point she was in the beginning stages of a heart transplant, but this summer she was doing so well she participated in a walkathon for charity! She has learned more about low-sodium diets than most nurses I know. She continues to be my hero for her fortitude and determination to be a good mama to her children.

We have been truly blessed. We had a nurse who followed the nursing journals and paid attention to research. We had doctors and a hospital that participated in a research study that would change our lives forever. And we had the Man upstairs who saw fit to let everyone survive intact. But that is not the end of the story . . .

Ironically, I was given a chance to "pay it forward" when a student at the college where I teach suffered the same type of full arrest. I was summoned to the room and performed CPR along with a coworker. The student was given the same hypothermic treatment and survived. It is only one month later, and she has already returned to her job. And next month, she plans to reenroll in her classes and finish the program. Now that's the end of the story . . . or is it?

EBP Pearl

Be vigilant, be innovative, be a positive deviant, and NEVER take "I CAN'T" for an answer!

This Is What We Do . . .

−Kathleen M. Lamaute, EdD, FNP Bc, CNE-A Bc, CNE
Associate Professor Division of Nursing
Molloy College, Rockville Centre, New York

It was 1992, and I was working as the manager of an electrophysiology department in a cardiac center. It was my responsibility to do routine pacemaker and implanted cardioverter defibrillator (ICD) interrogations. I saw patients every 2 months for their ICD check. I knew all my patients well. I knew their families, and I knew their routines. I also ran a support group for patients with implanted defibrillators that enabled me to help my patients transition into having and understanding their arrhythmia and their device.

At the time, it was standard education to inform patients that they could not be around large magnets because they would deactivate their defibrillator. I had a very nice patient who had to transfer the operation of his business (a junkyard that uses a large magnetic crane) to his son because the risk of deactivating the ICD was too great if he continued to work. He came regularly for his device check and seemed to adjust very well to the device and the follow-up care.

One day he and his wife came in for a routine device check, and I could tell something was wrong. I asked them what was going on, and they confided in me that their son was diagnosed with leukemia and was no longer able to run the business. They were trying to deal with their son's diagnosis as well as the loss of income and the family business.

I felt that I had to do something. I checked the literature thoroughly, and although it was clear that avoidance of magnetic fields was an important restriction given to all patients, I could not find anything that had specific measurements or scientific-based recommendations related to distance. What I did find out was that magnetic fields dropped significantly with small distances.

I called the manufacturer of the ICD and asked them if they could give me a device that would not fire (deliver a shock), but would "beep" just like all their devices beeped when they were deactivated by a magnet. I explained why I wanted to do this, and they were very cooperative. They sent out a representative with just such a device and with a gaussmeter to help me measure the magnetic field.

I called my patient and had him meet me at his junkyard. I brought the rigged device into the junkyard, stood by the crane, had the operator turn on the crane and I got into the cab of the operating crane. The device did not go off. I walked around outside of the crane while the magnet was turned on and I was able to go within 6 feet before the device beeped that it was deactivated. I repeated this a few times just to make sure the device behaved in a consistent manner.

After carefully collecting the observational data, we managed to identify a safe way for this patient to continue working at his junkyard as long as he followed specific safe distance measurements. I also arranged for him to come in for a device check more frequently just to make sure that his device was not inadvertently deactivated. I remember that visit to the junkyard clearly. It was almost Thanksgiving and it was very cold. When I finished testing the device with the crane and told him the results, he hugged me for a long time, and then he cried. I have never received a thank-you that was this touching

This was evidence-based nursing. This was seeing a patient with a problem and thinking critically about what I could do to help. This is what we do everyday as nurses. My patient's distress prompted me to go to the evidence that supported the recommendation that he avoid magnetic fields completely. I found it to be not complete and somewhat unreliable, which brought me to generating real-life evidence (i.e., internal evidence). I was able to collect my own data that led to a new recommendation for my patient. It made me wonder how many other patients there were who were like mine. How many people were given the recommendation to quit their jobs or change their lives because of magnetic fields? I realized that this story needed to be told. I wrote it up as a case study and submitted it to the *American Journal of Critical Care*. It was accepted and published in October 1993. This was true evidence-based practice, which not only looks for answers to new issues but calls into question established ones. In this case, it was the internal evidence (generated from practice data) that drove the recommendation and improved the patient outcome.

EBP Pearl

Accepted norms are not sacred. Always look for ways to improve practice, always question, and don't forget the best answer you have available might be in the data you collect about your own practice

The Traveling Journal Club

–Marion G. Mann, MSN, RN, CNS-BC
Expert Evidence-Based Practice Mentor
Baptist Medical Center, Nassau, Fernandina Beach, Florida

Journal club participation at our hospital was at an all-time low. Nurses complained that they didn't have time to participate while they were working and didn't want to come in on their day off. While trying to solve the problem and infuse a little enthusiasm, I noticed some nurses participating in various activities online, and I realized that a solution was right there in front of me. Technology! Over the next year, the Traveling Journal Club grew from a pilot at our small hospital to a system implementation for the entire health system of five hospitals and a home health agency.

The Traveling Journal Club (TJC) is an electronic journal club. Facilitators work with me (the Expert EBP Mentor) to choose an appropriate article by using the first four steps of EBP. Their desire to facilitate a journal club is acknowledged as a spirit of inquiry. After we have established their interests, they create a PICOT question, followed by a search for the best evidence. Then through critical appraisal, they can choose an article that represents the best evidence related to their inquiry. Nurses who are looking for opportunities to fulfill the requirements for their Clinical Ladder can use this tool while learning the EBP process. For some, it is a springboard for choosing an EBP project that can lead to clinical practice changes and/or research. After the facilitator sees their name "in lights" on the website, sometimes it encourages them to continue to showcase their work through presentations at their unit and system nursing councils. This often leads to submissions to conferences for poster and/or podium presentations.

For those who participate in the TJC, it is very convenient and fun. Entry is through the intranet portal for the hospital system. Each TJC has a home page with access to the article and the discussion board. After they have read the article and discussed it, they can complete a test and evaluation to receive 2 continuing education units (CEUs). Because it is online, the CEUs are sent directly to the CE broker for the board of nursing for our state. Because nurses are required to complete 20 CEUs per licensure period, this perk makes the TJC very popular among nurses.

Finding new and innovative ways to advance the EBP process is important to changing the paradigm. Health care is fast-paced and using technology is a valuable tool, especially for the new generation of nurses who have had technology at their fingertips since birth. Having the option to participate online 24/7 also increases participation by allowing nurses to choose a time that works with their schedule.

EBP Pearl

Innovation facilitates integration of EBP!

Helping Veterans Own Their Health: A Simple Evidence-Based Solution

–Sonya Myers, LPN
Primary Care University Drive
Veterans Health Administration Pittsburgh Healthcare System, Pittsburgh, Pennsylvania

Our team in the VA Primary Care comprises several highly motivated, challenge-driven, dedicated, and educated LPNs, including Evie, Danya, Sheila, Dawn, Debbie, David, Trina, and me. Our team is led by a nurse manager, Christin, who encourages, acknowledges, and rewards individual and collective contributions, efforts, and accomplishments that demonstrate a highly functioning team. During 2009, Primary Care had consistently fallen below the threshold for completion of colorectal screening in their patient population. It is expected that a veteran who meets criteria will be screened for colorectal cancer either through completion of a colonoscopy, sigmoidoscopy, or fecal occult blood testing, and this screening will be documented. Because this was a Veterans Health Administration (VHA) performance measure, greater emphasis was placed on meeting this measure. Our team was aware of the importance of early detection and prevention through screening, but we wondered whether or not the same was true for our veterans.

The call for an action plan was presented to the professional practice council and the challenge began. Part of our team gathered preliminary data collection and analysis to identify barriers that prevented screenings from being completed. Our results indicated that our veteran patients were most reluctant to have a colonoscopy for screening and, instead, opted to perform fecal occult blood testing. However, most of our patients were reluctant to complete this test at home and send by mail because it seemed embarrassing to them. After our team identified this main barrier, we had to be creative in getting the patient to return the stool cards. This prompted us to benchmark with other VAs to determine best practices that were successful in achieving this goal. We also conducted searches in the literature to discover a viable evidence-based solution.

Our benchmarking combined with the search for research evidence determined the most effective way to ensure completion and return of the fecal cards was to provide follow-up phone calls to veterans who had not returned their cards. The research evidence indicated that when veterans received a call that reeducated them and clarified the importance of this screening, they were more likely to complete the test and return the cards. The plan was that a veteran would be administered a fecal card packet, and it had to be mailed and received in the lab within 2 weeks. If the card was not returned within 2 weeks, one of our team would call the veteran to follow-up. Reeducation was provided as needed, or if cards were destroyed or misplaced, then a new set was mailed. If another 2 weeks passed and the cards were still not registered into the system, our team would mail out a reminder letter that we created and include a new set of cards. With implementation of this new, evidence-based process, our team experienced a slow and gradual improvement in the return rate of fecal occult blood testing cards. Early in 2009, our second quarter performance for returning fecal cards was at 73%, with a goal of 79%. By the end of 2009, our return rate had improved beyond the threshold to a sustained 86%.

This improvement not only contributed to the health and well-being of our veterans, but it also created a culture in which the expected norm was for veterans to return their fecal cards or they would be *hunted down until they did*—all in good fun, of course. An added benefit was that physicians noticed a decrease in the need for veterans to require additional education to promote compliance with their return of the cards. Our team was recognized and rewarded with a pizza party and an unexpected, yet much appreciated, group cash award from our fearless leader and biggest cheerleader, our nurse manager! Our team participated in our hospital's Magnet Munch-n-Mingle event, creating an innovative poster presentation that replicated life-size versions of stool cards and supplied food that resembled feces (brownies and fudge) and "Golytely" juice to disseminate how our evidence-based solution had been successful in improving outcomes. Through this initiative, our team not only improved the quality of care for our veterans, but we also overcame challenges that made us stronger as a team and had fun improving outcomes through the use of the evidence-based practice (EBP) process.

EBP Pearl

Innovation goes hand-in-hand with EBP.

A Better Quality of Life Through the Use of Hip Protectors

–*Emma C. Pittman, MS, BSN, RN,*
Community Living Center, Liberty City
Orlando VA Medical Center, Orlando, Florida

"Jake" was a tall, handsome man with well-groomed, silvery-gray hair, quick with a smile and a greeting, and he loved to share his war stories. Charming and respectful, he was proud that he could still take care of himself, with just a little assistance and direction from the staff of Liberty City, the locked Dementia Unit in our Community Living Center at the Orlando VA Medical Center. He enjoyed participating in Liberty City's group activities, always polite and cooperative with the staff and congenial with his fellow residents.

Unfortunately, all that changed in just seconds in mid-2008 when Jake fell and fractured his hip—a mishap that occurs all too often with the elderly. Restricted to a wheelchair for most of the time after his fall, he gradually deteriorated; we watched as he became less social and more dependent on staff for assistance. Easily agitated, he became less cooperative as his medical problems increased, and his physical condition deteriorated until he passed away. His transformation from a vibrant soul to a shell of the previous man with little vitality was heartbreaking to watch. Our nurses and other staff become very attached to our residents of Liberty City—these veterans who have given so much to us—and it can be very depressing to watch the light within them fade away.

After seeing what happened to Jake, we were determined to do everything we could to prevent a reoccurrence of such suffering. Seeing the profound impact that a hip fracture had on someone as full of life as Jake was particularly disheartening to the staff of Liberty City, and his deterioration spurred us on to seek a solution to prevent any similar tragedies for these American heroes. Even before Jake's fall, we had implemented an evidence-based prevention method for fall complications—hip protectors. However, we faced some initial difficulties in their use and some reluctance by patients to accept them. Hip protectors are designed to protect those areas vulnerable to injury in a fall, but both staff and patients were initially hesitant to use them. However, over time, the design of hip protectors has markedly improved, and now they are much more customized in types, styles, and sizes to fit the individual needs of the user. Through consultation and collaboration with the VISN 8 Patient Safety Center on the use of hip protectors, the Liberty City staff have been educated on their value and correct usage, and now, as part of the admission process, an RN will discuss hip protector use with each resident and the family, explaining that the use of hip protectors is a standard practice for our unit. This communication from the beginning of the resident's stay stresses our commitment to the resident's safety and the critical importance of using hip protectors, both day and night.

Choices for the resident are maximized through the offering of a variety of types and styles of hip protectors that can be used in undergarments, shorts, and long pants. Several pairs are provided to the resident, marked with a date of initial use and laundered by the staff. A record is kept of each resident's hip protectors and their daily use, and the resident and the family are educated as to their use. The hip protectors are monitored to insure proper condition.

As a result of this proactive program, since mid-2008, we have had no more "Jakes" resulting from hip fractures. Liberty City has a 90–95% rate of daily usage of hip protectors in its 40-bed unit and is considered to be a best practice in the use of hip protectors. In May 2010, this unit was awarded the VISN 8 Patient Safety Center of Inquiry Best Practice Award for Falls Injury Prevention. This successful program has resulted in significant reductions in cost, injuries, disabilities, institutionalization, and diminished quality of life for veterans.

Unfortunately, aged, frail residents will suffer falls, despite the best preventative measures. In 2009, Liberty City residents, with an average census of 35 residents, experienced 45 falls. Potentially, any or all of those falls could have resulted in a hip fracture for the resident. The average cost for hospitalization resulting from a hip fracture is approximately $30,000. The total approximate cost of about 260 hip protectors used in 2009 was $16,996. The cost savings in preventing just one hip fracture is dramatic.

Most important is the veterans' improved functioning, independence, safety, and quality of life that is sustained because of prevented hip fractures. Liberty City is an activity-based community, designed to provide the best possible quality of life for each veteran, and the increased use of hip protectors has become a critical factor in ensuring their quality of care and safety. A significant bonus has been the increased sense of satisfaction that our Liberty City staff have in their service to the veterans. Our work satisfaction levels have increased as the stress felt over patient safety has decreased, and this decreased stress level has helped to sustain a 0% staff turnover for the past 2 years.

Hip protectors will not prevent falls by elderly patients, but they will greatly reduce the risks of significant hip injuries that negatively impact the quality of life for our residents. The low cost of hip protectors is more than offset by the enhanced quality of life that our resident veterans maintain, as well as the increased peace of mind and satisfaction of our staff and the residents' families. Not seeing the diminishing of any more "Jakes" makes all the difference in the world!

EBP Pearl

Think innovation, think evaluation, think change . . . THINK EBP!

Harmonica Playing: An Easy and Fun Way to Improve Quality of Life in Patients with COPD

–*Sharon Miller, BSN, RN, CCRN*
Cardiopulmonary Rehabilitation Nurse
Mid Coast Hospital, Brunswick, Maine

I began my nursing career over 25 years ago in the intensive care unit and cardiac/pulmonary rehabilitation unit in a small community hospital in a rural state in New England. Although I am passionate about the specialty in which I practice, I have recently felt I needed something challenging to help stimulate my career. I heard about a Clinical Scholars Program at a nearby hospital. I remember being interested in research when I was getting my baccalaureate degree, but thought you needed to work in a laboratory at a university to conduct research. At the time, my hospital was applying for the Magnet Recognition Program; therefore, my nursing colleagues encouraged me to take the Clinical Scholars Program. Because of budgetary constraints that all hospitals are enduring during these tough economic times, my director wanted me to write a proposal as to why I wanted to take the Clinical Scholars Program and what I hoped to gain from attending. My director had not practiced nursing in a number of years, which added to the challenges of trying to explain to him the importance of learning the skill set needed to achieve evidence-based practice (EBP).

The Clinical Scholars Program is a series of seven workshops that teaches nurses and other health care practitioners the EBP process and the conduct of research. This program consists of didactic lectures on a variety of topics, including "Research Designs," "Critical Appraisal of the Scientific Evidence," "Introduction to Statistics," and many others. Each workshop afternoon was devoted to participants being divided into smaller clinical groups where they received group and individual support for project development.

I enjoyed the program because it was a well-organized learning experience guiding us through starting a research project and beyond. Mentors helped support the learning process. In these groups, we brainstormed ideas with nurses working in other hospitals around the state. You could almost palpate the excitement growing with the synergistic energy for the birth of the various research projects.

My idea to study harmonica playing as a means of pulmonary rehabilitation in chronic obstructive pulmonary disease (COPD) patients came from a respiratory therapist with whom I work. He told me that he had heard about this, and it captured my interest. I decided to start teaching harmonica playing with my maintenance cardiac and pulmonary rehab group that meets three times per week. I had been playing the harmonica with them for over a year when I started the Clinical Scholars Program.

I wanted my first research project to be seamless (don't we all!), and my mentor encouraged me to think outside the box. I decided to focus my research project on the harmonica playing I had previously introduced to my patients, but had no data to support its benefits. I began conducting a literature search. It quickly became apparent that no literature related to COPD patients playing the harmonica existed. I decided I really wanted to do this research because, anecdotally, I had noticed that one of my patients would take his oxygen off so I could check his O_2 saturation. It was 92% prior to playing the harmonica, but after playing the harmonica for 10 minutes, his O_2 saturations were 95%. I did several spot checks, and his oxygen saturations always improved, which added to my excitement about doing this project.

Thus began my scholarly journey. My research project was entitled "A Comparison of COPD Patients' Quality of Life Using the Harmonica as a Means of Pulmonary Rehabilitation." It was a randomized controlled study with a control group and an experimental (harmonica playing) group. My hypothesis was that playing the harmonica was an effective tool for clearing the airways of mucous, thereby improving oxygenation and leading to less oxygen use, a decreased need for antibiotics, emergency department visits, hospitalizations, and improvements in quality of life scores.

With assistance and support from the mentors of the program, I performed a power analysis and determined that I needed 12 subjects in each group to determine statistical significance. The research nurse coordinator assisted with writing the proposal, the IRB application, and other aspects of getting my study off the ground.

At the time of this writing, I have completed patient enrollment, and my data is being analyzed. I am anxious to see the analysis from my study and am hoping that it has proven to be a benefit to patients with COPD. I can say that I have had some very positive comments from the patients in the harmonica group who really enjoyed learning a musical instrument.

One of my patients was a 65-year-old woman who had never played a musical instrument, but by the end of the program, she had learned to play 10 to 12 songs. She was going to teach her grandchild how to play and was excited to play it with him. To see the smile on her face and her enthusiasm filled my heart with joy. A few other comments from patients were as follows: "Had not played the harmonica in many years. I enjoyed this session, and I have come to understand that breathing through the harmonica has done my lungs good. I will continue to do so, thank you all." "Sharon is enthusiastic and encouraging. I believe that playing the harmonica helps improve my breathing. I plan to continue." "First of all, I must say that I enjoyed this study very much. It helped me to know how to breathe properly. The harmonica was a good tool for this, I think. I looked forward to the sessions and the instructions given by Mrs. Miller, RN."

These anonymous comments have made me feel really good about the work that I am doing as a cardiopulmonary rehabilitation nurse, restoring my commitment to providing a compassionate caring practice, based on evidence. I think this story of how attending a series of evidence-based practice workshops, learning how to conduct research, completing a study, and applying it to practice will dismiss any misconceptions about research not being fun!

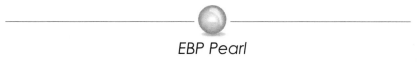

EBP Pearl

Thinking outside of the box as "positive deviants" can result in innovative EBP changes that improve patient outcomes.

Flashcards: A Human Touch

–Liliana G. Suchicital, BSN, RN, CBN
Inova Fair Oaks Hospital
Fairfax, Virginia

As a nurse clinician for more than 30 years, I have practiced in many settings and have witnessed many drastic changes in the profession. I still remember the needles with glass syringes and the autoclaves used to sterilize them. Thanks to technology, glass syringes are history. In fact, across the board in nursing, new and better methods for many of our practices have evolved, and as a result, patients are receiving more efficient, evidence-based, safer, and individualized care than ever before.

However, for a patient lying sick in the room of a hospital, no matter how highly credentialed the hospital, all of the high-tech hospital equipment and well-trained staff in the world will not matter if the patient and staff cannot communicate.

In this age of innovation in health care, nurses must recognize that our primary role as communicator is one part of the profession that has not changed. In fact, we cannot provide excellent care without excellent communication.

As nurses, we are integral to providing care to our patients and, in many cases, their families as well. We are the bridge that supports many other disciplines in providing holistic patient care; we are the strongest link between the patient and the rest of the team. We carry out physicians' orders and coordinate services with other members of the team, such as radiologists, physical therapists, laboratory technicians, and discharge managers. For many of us, a majority of our shifts are spent explaining, questioning, listening, and teaching, all to deliver the best individualized care plan for each patient. As part of evidence-based practice (EBP), we must integrate our clinical expertise to implement innovations in patient care.

When you recognize the importance of communication in the hospital setting, it becomes easy to see how a patient with a different cultural heritage or ethnicity who speaks a different language could feel totally lost in our American hospital system. A language barrier leaves patients dependent on others to convey their needs. This dependence increases patients' sense of helplessness and loss of control. These patients have real fear because they might not understand what is happening, or they might be terrified we will not understand their needs. At the same time, inability to talk to and understand a patient only adds to the bedside nurse's sense of frustration. In addition, on top of the patient's fear and nurse's frustration are important patient safety issues that are compromised when loved ones—many times children—are asked to act as interpreters.

Inova Health Systems is in Fairfax, Virginia, which is home to one million residents. It is one of the most diverse counties in the United States. The challenge for Inova is to provide quality care to all residents, regardless of their ethnicities or cultural backgrounds. In 2006, 26.8% of our population was foreign-born, and 32.9% of our residents over age five spoke a language other than English at home. A minimum of six languages are spoken by the nurses and another six different languages by assistive personnel.

With patients from around the world visiting its hospitals every day, Inova has recognized that patient communication must be a top priority. The company has instituted specific interpreter training courses—in many languages—for clinical professionals. These certified interpreters are easily accessible in person or via telephone, which is an evidence-based practice commonly used in many hospitals today.

However, as a direct care nurse, I have observed that the interpreter program can fall short. When interpretation services are not readily available because interpreters might be busy on different units, patients might have to wait longer than reasonably expected to relay their needs. Similarly, when the interpreter phone line gives a busy signal, a simple need might go unattended. In truth, the time-consuming chore of seeking out an interpreter or dialing the language line might prevent nurses from using these services. Thus, care is compromised.

The bottom line is that patients who are in pain or need to use the restroom should not have to wait for help just because they do not speak English. So, I began looking for a way to change the way we practice.

As a certified interpreter in English and Spanish, I knew I needed a simple tool to help me reach my non-English-speaking patients. Flashcards, I thought. Flashcards are a favorite of educators; they are easy to develop and use. I decided to give flashcards a try.

I created a series of flashcards using our five most common foreign languages: Spanish, Korean, Chinese, Vietnamese, and Hindi. I wrote our basic tasks/questions including patients' comfort (pain, hot/cold, nausea); nutrition; mobility; toileting; and safety issues in both English and the foreign language, one task per card. They are written in simple terms, in as few words as possible, so they can be understood by our patients even with basic reading skills. The cards do not include any medical terminology. Each card also has an illustration alongside the words for our patients who cannot read. Finally, the cards are laminated, clipped together like mini-flip charts, and stored in the central nursing station. We now even use English cards for our English-speaking patients who because of their medical condition (such as jaw surgery) can use the flashcard pictures instead of constantly writing notes for simple requests.

These flashcards are not intended to replace the phones or interpreters for complex patient/family education, assessments, or in-depth questions and answers. The cards are meant to be a quick, easy tool to meet a patient's basic needs.

Nurses on my unit found the cards helpful in their daily care of non-English speakers; they facilitated prompt, stress-free care. The cards also helped nurses assess whether more extensive communication was needed via the language phone or interpreter. By using the flashcards, patients could communicate quickly and get more comfortable quickly, which improved their confidence in our care, increased their satisfaction, and perhaps, most importantly, decreased their stress.

I once had a patient, Mrs. V, an elderly Mandarin-speaking woman, who was admitted to the surgical unit after bowel surgery. When I met her, she was on a clear liquid diet, and she was working hard toward a speedy recovery so she could go home with her daughter. Her daughter was concerned because she felt uncomfortable leaving her mother alone in the hospital, even when her mother had the interpreter phone at the bedside. On the other hand, one of the daughter's children was about to start kindergarten and Mrs. V's daughter needed to be at home to help the child get ready for school. I explained the use of the flashcards to her, and she in turn explained them to her mother.

After a couple hours, Mrs. V. called me into her room. She looked at me calmly, and with a shy smile showed me one of the flashcards. It was the one that read, "I passed gas." I nodded to let her know I that understood what she was trying to say, and I reassessed her bowel sounds. They were strong and present in all four quadrants. I was in the process of waiting for her doctor to call me back, so I could address Mrs. V's progress with him. However, she called me in again, and when I arrived to her room, she was sitting in the recliner chair almost giggling with another flashcard in her hand. This time she showed me the one that said, "I moved my bowels." She looked confident and self-assured because she had this tool to make me aware of her progress. This is when it hit me: the impact of the language and the pictures on these simple flashcards could make a real difference in a patient's care.

At the news of the improving bowel function, Mrs. V's physician promptly advanced her diet to soft, and Mrs. V got to enjoy a tasty soft-diet dinner before food services closed that day. The flashcards allowed her to tell me something early in the day that otherwise she likely would have communicated through her daughter late that evening.

Her daughter, whom I saw just before the end of my shift, was grateful to know her mother's basic needs were met. I felt empowered, knowing my nursing intervention impacted Mrs. V's quality of care and shortened the length of her stay. The next morning she was discharged and back home with her beloved family.

I was satisfied to see my flashcards worked. I submitted the project to the hospital's "Fair Oaks Best Idea Contest" and was proud to receive one of the awards. However, I won't stop there; I want to continually work to advance the art of nursing. Currently, I am preparing a protocol for a human caring study that will analyze the impact of human touch through pictures in patient care. Even after 30 years in nursing, I know so many practices can be rethought and revised, all to improve our patients' outcomes.

EBP Pearl

Ideas that are implemented are innovations that can improve the quality of health care and patient outcomes; so go forth and innovate.

3

Incorporating Patient Preferences and Clinician Expertise in Evidence-Based Practice

A patient's (or family's) preferences and values along with a clinician's expertise are important components of evidence-based practice that too often get overlooked and not factored into decisions about patient care. It is so important to remember that patients are not just statistics; they often do not perform the way studies predict they will. Therefore, it is imperative to seek out and listen to the preferences and values of your patients and family members, provide them with the best evidence to inform their preferences, and to actively involve them routinely in care decisions. Clinicians are the key to integrating best evidence with internal evidence gathered from patient data and patients' preferences and values. It is important to recognize the impact that your clinical experience and expertise makes on health care outcomes.

This chapter contains stories that will enhance your understanding of the importance of including patient-family preferences and your clinical expertise as an integral part of evidence-based practice. Place yourself in these individuals' shoes, try to feel what they feel, and consider how you can make a change toward best practice or foster change in your colleagues to keep patient preferences and values, as well as clinical expertise, part of daily decision-making. This will help you stay true to the core reasons that you chose your profession—caring for individuals to make a positive impact in their health and lives.

Kaylin's Story: Australian Dream Trip Turned Nightmare

–Bernadette Mazurek Melnyk, PhD, RN, CPNP/PMHNP, FNAP, FAAN
Dean and Distinguished Foundation Professor in Nursing
Arizona State University College of Nursing & Health Innovation, Phoenix, Arizona

My husband, John, and our youngest daughter, Kaylin, who was 8 years old at the time, were so excited about our dream trip to Australia. We'd long talked about visiting Australia, especially the Australian outback. I was scheduled to make a presentation at an international conference in Brisbane, so we decided it would be the perfect time for our long-awaited dream to become reality. We decided to first visit New Zealand before heading on to Australia to see some wonderful sites there. Our trip's first layover was in the Los Angeles airport, where we ate dinner, and Kaylin enjoyed an ice cream sundae. She was the picture of health when we left Los Angeles and was so excited to be going to the land of koala bears. However, approximately 3 hours from New Zealand, Kaylin awakened me from a deep sleep to let me know that she was feeling sick, specifically saying that her "belly hurt." I felt her forehead, and it was obvious that she had a fever. Then within an hour, she started vomiting. The pediatric nurse practitioner (PNP) mom in me suspected early appendicitis. The pattern of fever and abdominal pain preceding vomiting were the classic symptoms for appendicitis that I had taught my PNP students for many years. I woke my husband to let him know that Kaylin was sick and that I suspected early appendicitis. He was in disbelief as she was healthy when we left Los Angeles. John also was convinced that this was a "gastrointestinal (GI) bug" that he had experienced 4 days earlier.

Kaylin continued to vomit intermittently for the rest of the flight to New Zealand. I knew she had to be seen for a thorough evaluation. After landing, we went immediately to a 24-hour medical facility where I conveyed my concern about early appendicitis to the pediatrician who evaluated her. After examining her and running a few lab tests, the physician decided that she just had a GI virus and we could take her to our hotel. The pediatrician kept emphasizing that Kaylin did not have abdominal rebound, which is a common sign of appendicitis. My husband looked at me like, "I knew it was just that GI bug," but something in my gut still gnawed at me and told me that there was more to Kaylin's illness.

After 48 hours, Kaylin's temperature dropped and she stopped all vomiting, so I was finally ready to admit that I had been the overprotective PNP mom. I must have palpated Kaylin's abdomen 10 times a day for those 2 days to reassure myself that she did not have appendicitis. I felt relieved as we left New Zealand for Sydney, Australia.

We spent 4 days in Sydney, touring the most common attractions. Kaylin did not seem her normal self. She was even complacent about seeing koala bears at the zoo, which was unusual because that was all that she talked about before we left for our trip. During the time we were in Sydney, Kaylin was without fever and did not complain any further about abdominal pain. However, she was pale, lacked an appetite, walked a little humped over, and was not her energetic self. My husband and I rationalized that it was the aftermath of a bad GI virus.

After 4 days, we flew to a place called Ayers Rock in the Australian outback. The second day there, we went to the Sounds of Silence dinner. Being in the Australian outback, under the grand sky with a view of the magnificent rock, listening to didgeridoo music, and watching one of the most incredible sunsets ever seen was awe-inspiring. After dinner, under a host of stars, an astrologist gave us an overview of the star constellations. Kaylin still lacked her appetite and literally fell asleep on the table at dinner. I was still concerned about her, but my husband continued to remind me that she was not only jet-lagged, but recovering from a nasty GI flu.

We were to fly from Ayers Rock to Cairns, Australia, the next morning. During the night, John and I were awakened by the sound of groans coming from Kaylin in her sleep. I felt her forehead, and she was burning up with fever. As I woke up Kaylin to take her temperature (I always traveled with a stock of needed supplies and medications), my mind raced back to her symptoms over the past week and I now knew, deep down, that an appendicitis was missed. I was convinced Kaylin's appendix had ruptured, and now we were into a serious medical situation with an abscess. We took the next flight out of Ayers Rock, and as soon as we landed, took Kaylin to another medical facility. The physician there was very good and also was concerned about a ruptured appendix. Kaylin's blood work came back, and, as I had feared, it showed a 33,000 white blood cell count, 92% neutrophils, and 36 bands/stabs. We rushed to the emergency department of the public hospital in Cairns, knowing we had a very serious medical situation.

We were in the emergency room at the public hospital for hours. Kaylin was examined by multiple physicians and a surgeon, who had her jumping up and down on her right foot, assuring us that this was not an abdominal problem because she was able to do that task. More blood tests and cultures were performed, and after hours, we were told that we could take her back to the hotel as it was just a virus, even though I was insistent that she had a ruptured appendix. I kept telling the physicians that the severe shift to the left in Kaylin's lab work indicated a severe bacterial, not viral infection. I begged the physicians for an MRI or ultrasound of her abdomen, but they would not perform the test. Finally, after some time of pleading to admit Kaylin to the hospital, they admitted her to the pediatric unit. The head nurse later told me that she was labeled a "soft admission," but they were admitting her to the hospital because she had a stressed out nurse mom from the United States who was insistent upon her admission.

Throughout the night and during the entire next day, Kaylin was evaluated by six or seven physicians. I told the same story to each physician, insisting that she had a ruptured appendix and was now into an abscess. Kaylin was looking worse to me—her fever remained at 104 degrees, she had tachycardia out of proportion to her fever, and she was starting to look septic. I was a former pediatric intensive care unit nurse and was keenly aware of early signs and symptoms of sepsis. After pleading with multiple physicians, asking them for an ultrasound of her abdomen, the last physician finally agreed to the test. An ultrasound was performed, which revealed a huge abscess from a ruptured appendix in Kaylin's abdomen.

One of the public surgeons came in to communicate the results of the ultrasound to us. He said that the best treatment was to place Kaylin on IV triple dose antibiotics *for six weeks* in hopes that her body would wall the abscess off, and then, an elective surgery could be performed to remove it and what was left of the appendix. I was almost apoplectic as I knew that Kaylin would be septic in the next 24 hours if we did not take a more aggressive approach to treatment. I asked the surgeon for the evidence base behind his recommended treatment, and he could not give me a solid answer. As I was sobbing and so wishing we were at home at a hospital with physicians with whom I was familiar and who I believed would have listened to me, Kaylin's nurse said that, as an American, I could call for a consult from a private surgeon. I asked her to get us the best surgeon in town, which she did. I will never forget that pediatric nurse, because without her, Kaylin might have never made it home.

A couple of hours later, the private surgeon walked into the room. I had a good sense about him, right from the very beginning. After evaluating Kaylin, he told us that he needed to get her to the theater (operating room) immediately as she was full of infection and on the verge of sepsis. We breathed a sigh of relief. After more than a day of pleading with multiple physicians and asking for the evidence behind decisions that were being made, we finally had someone engaged in evidence-based decision-making.

Kaylin was in surgery for a few hours. By the time of surgery, she had full blown peritonitis and pelvic sepsis, but never did she have classic guarding that is seen with peritonitis. She was not the typical case of appendicitis because she had a retroverted appendix, so she did not have the classic "rebound" that is commonly seen in children with appendicitis. Because of her extensive infection, Kaylin's peritoneal cavity had to be flushed with saline for 2 solid hours. My husband and I were never so relieved as to see the surgeon emerge from the operating room and tell us that he believed Kaylin would have an extensive recovery, but that she would be alright.

Kaylin's recovery was indeed slow. She lost about 10 pounds, developed an ileus after surgery, and had extensive infection that was tough to resolve. After 2 weeks in the hospital, Kaylin finally recovered enough for us to take her back to our hotel. Because her abdomen was still distended, we could not fly home for another week. During her hospital stay, the surgeon who examined Kaylin in the emergency department came to see us and apologized profusely for missing the diagnosis earlier. Later that week, he conducted grand rounds and reviewed Kaylin's case with numerous physicians so that her atypical case of a ruptured appendix would not be missed again.

While Kaylin was in the hospital, a news story on television reported that a little girl had died of meningitis at the same hospital. I found myself wondering whether that mother, too, faced the same situation as we did in terms of advocating for her child with health care providers who did not listen intently and take her input seriously. As parents, we know our children best, but do not always have providers who listen keenly to what we have to offer. I reflected a lot on evidence-based practice while Kaylin was in the hospital and how her case was a prime example of how various elements of EBP were not taken into consideration.

After a few days back at the hotel, Kaylin's surgeon finally gave us permission to take Kaylin to the beautiful rain forest in Cairns. I will never forget riding the sky cab over the rain forest and taking a picture of my pale little girl, smiling from ear to ear, so happy to be out of the hospital. That picture of Kaylin still sits in our family room as a constant reminder of how blessed we were to have come through that Australian dream trip, turned nightmare. Although still quite weak, Kaylin beamed as she finally got a chance to have one of her dreams come true—to hold a koala bear.

After nearly 4 weeks in Australia, we landed in Los Angeles again. Kaylin was so happy to be back in the United States, saying that she never wanted to leave America again. John and I, too, were ecstatic that we were bringing our little girl back home. To this day, we are tremendously thankful for Kaylin's pediatric nurse and her surgeon. We ache for the parents who lose their children, especially when medicine goes awry and deaths or medical errors could have been prevented. We now know that one in 10 patients admitted to the hospital will experience a medical error. We also know that EBP, which integrates the best evidence with a clinician's expertise and patient's preferences and values, results in the highest quality, low-cost health care with the best patient outcomes. However, what often is not taught or emphasized enough in EBP is how to factor in a patient/family member's preferences or a clinician's expertise into the evidence-based decision-making process. It is my hope that our daughter Kaylin's story will help clinicians never forget to listen to and heed the wisdom/preferences of patient's or their family member's and to always listen to their clinical expertise when making the best evidence-based decisions about patient care. Through EBP and advocating for what we know is soundly based on the EBP process, we can avoid more complications and save more patient lives.

EBP Pearl

Always listen intently to your patients (and family members), taking into consideration their preferences/values and your own clinical expertise as part of the evidence-based decision-making process; it could very well save your patients' lives.

From the Other Side of the Bed

–Ellen Fineout-Overholt, PhD, RN, FNAP, FAAN
Clinical Professor & Director, Center for the Advancement of Evidence-Based Practice
Arizona State University, Phoenix, Arizona

This story is but one of many that underpin the passion that I have for practicing based on evidence— evidence from science, evidence from practice— blended with expertise and the patient and family preferences. Without fully incorporating patient preferences, it really isn't evidence-based practice. My dad and I had a close relationship that was based on discussion of world events and spiritual truths. He was my example of a "thinker" who had faith. I admired him greatly. My dad had his first heart attack around 1973. The mode of treatment then was strict bedrest and few visitors. After this event, he had a few bouts with angina, but nothing too serious.

In the summer of 1990, my parents and I went on vacation in the northeast United States and found ourselves in a predicament that left us wondering what would come next. Our car was stolen, and we had nothing to our name but the clothes on our backs and our wallets. My dad, in an attempt to thwart the deed, was injured to the point that he tore his rotator cuff and needed it repaired. After the surgery in December, he began to have difficulty breathing, especially at night. On x-ray, everything looked clear. His blood work appeared normal. The physicians caring for my dad had no answers. Later we found out that he had a perioperative myocardial infarction that was unknown to him, my mom, and me. This laid the foundation for what was to come.

One day in the late spring of 1991, I got the call that everyone dreads. My mom told me that my dad had complained of severe chest pain to the point that he wanted her to call 911. The failure of the system began at that point. The ambulance crew forced him to walk down the stairs in his home, and dropped him off the gurney on the way to the ambulance. When my mom told me this, I began thinking of the workload on his heart. After all, he called 911 because he was having chest pain. She told me that he had been taken to the emergency department (ED) where he had a respiratory and/or cardiac arrest. My mom is an American history teacher—I was glad she knew to tell me that much. I couldn't believe it— *MY DAD* had a cardiac arrest?! Mom told me that the ED team had resuscitated him, and he was now in an intensive care unit (ICU) on a ventilator. At the time, I lived 1,500 miles away from my parents. All I could do was pray that he wouldn't die before I could see him.

I arrived the next day to find my Dad extubated, but laboring to breathe. In my desperate attempt to connect, I asked him, "Do you know who I am?" He looked at me as if I was crazy, and said, "You're Ellen!" Sometimes we must appear very foolish to our patients! At the time, I had been a critical care nurse for 14 years and had seen many patients die of complications after they entered the health care system. Now my dad was in the health care system, had arrested, was laboring to breathe, and was hemodynamically unstable. They had inserted an intra-aortic balloon (IAB) after his arrest. He was on renal dose dopamine. I feared the worst and prayed for the best to happen.

The medical team believed it was in Dad's best interest to re-intubate him that evening. When I went in to see him, he had white frothy secretions in his endotracheal tube. The nurse had his back to us and seemed engrossed in what he was doing. I instinctively reached down, turned on the 100% oxygen, and suctioned Dad out with the in-line suction device. Some of you are cringing as you read this. Put yourself in my shoes. Granted, maybe I ought to have asked, but emotions sometimes cloud judgement. It was my dad, and he was struggling to breathe. I acted out of instinct and experience, and it happened only once. My actions were visibly frowned upon, but no one discussed them with me. The nurses were apprehensive about my role in caring for my dad. They were hesitant to let me review the chart. Even the physicians were defensive when I quoted my dad's "numbers" (e.g., cardiac index) to them and asked their thoughts and plans. The communication was breaking down, and my dad was getting worse. There were no support mechanisms to intervene for my family.

The next event was an embolus from the IAB. The health care team indicated that my dad might die when the IAB was removed, so we filed in to say goodbye before they took him for an embolectomy. The IAB was removed without incident, and the surgery went fine. This was the first clue to me that perhaps gaps existed not only in the communication with our family, but among those caring for Dad. Something wasn't measuring up—they expected him to die, and he did not. I began to wonder and pursue information about his other systems besides his heart, but I had to ask the provider who was "in charge" of that system. Seeking out each provider became a difficult endeavor and an emotional drain on me. My family looked to me to provide information and to try to piece together the responses to treatment that we were seeing. How do you, as a family member and a nurse, answer questions like, "They thought he was going to die, but he did fine. Why don't they know what is going on?"

Eventually, my dad went for bypass grafts because they still thought his primary problem was his cardiovascular disease. He was moved to a surgical ICU. The nurses in this ICU promptly told me, "You are welcome to visit your father, but you won't be allowed to participate in the kinds of actions you did in the other ICU, such as suctioning." There seemed to be an adversarial relationship between the nursing staff and me, even before my dad was admitted. I didn't like this approach by the nursing staff, but was too emotionally exhausted to deal with it. I was too busy trying to figure out what was happening with my dad. I was poring over physiology and critical care books and was trying to explain his blood values, the treatment plans, outcomes, and dynamics of the health care team to my family. The medical team had minimal communication — less than daily contacts— with my family. Subsequently in the next week, my dad was extubated and re-intubated again, was on continuous arterial venous hemofiltration, was on multiple vasopressor drips, and had become unresponsive without an explanation. Then, he became septic—my worst nightmare—and there was nothing I could do about it.

Then and now evidence exists that supports the role of an ethics team (now a whole specialty exists, called palliative care) that can help families and patients make decisions around the designation of Do Not Resuscitate (DNR). During the entire hospitalization, no mention was made of an ethics team or any other support to help us as a family make decisions. Decision-making for us was difficult. Knowing that my father could die, knowing the impact that loss would have on my family, and understanding the impact of my role in telling them this information made the emotional burden on me tremendous. My father deteriorated in front of our eyes, and the medical team rarely came to discuss care with us. Because I am the only health care professional in my family, it fell on my shoulders to explain that my dad was dying. It would have been wonderful to have an advocate to inform and support our decision-making.

Ultimately, we as a family had a conference with ourselves and decided to wean Levophed and dopamine, not to initiate any other measures, and to designate my dad as a DNR. We received a lot of flack from the medical team, especially the attending physician. (Sometimes we get caught up in our work and forget that those for whom we care need just a bit of our time and attention.) I walked with this physician to the cardiac catheterization lab to discuss with him the choice of DNR for my dad, as he offered me no other options for when or where to have this sensitive conversation. Unfortunately, the person who was supposed to be taking care of my dad was consistently unavailable, noncommunicative, and did not include our family in caring for Dad. The nurses seemed aware of the situation, but none intervened on our behalf.

These events occurred over 20 years ago, but we know that sometimes this still happens today. Given the plethora of evidence that supports the role of the family in caring for a loved one who is critically ill, we as nurses must consider current practice. It is important to keep the outcome in mind; including families who want to participate in care of their loved ones, even if it means an uncomfortable change in our practice, will improve the outcomes for *that* family.

Within 24 hours of weaning the drips, Dad died. Many thoughts went through my mind, like: Since Dad was unresponsive, did he die peacefully? Would he have died more peacefully if we were at his side more often than 15 minutes every 2 hours? I will never have answers to those questions, but I know that I know that receiving care by clinicians who are practicing based on evidence, including patient preferences, and focusing on outcome will make a difference in the experiences of patients and families who may find themselves in similar situations.

EBP Pearl

Patient and family preferences are paramount to successful outcomes in health care!

The Card

–Frannie Beth Hibbs-Concaugh, RN, PCRN
Oncology Nurse of the Year 2010, Tampa General Hospital Nurse of the Year 2010 (Acute Care)
Tampa General Hospital, Tampa, Florida

I will never forget my first week working in the chemotherapy clinic here at Tampa General Hospital. I was a bit nervous, not knowing what to expect and wanting to take advantage of every minute possible during this learning experience. I knew that this week was my opportunity to ask questions, learn, administer medication, enhance my clinical skills, and prepare myself for inpatient chemotherapy administration during my current shift assignment (night shift). On nights, you do not have the advantage of a unit-based chemotherapy pharmacist available for questions and other perks that come with daylight operating hours. So I was set to tackle this week with due diligence, making the most of my time in the clinic. What I failed to anticipate this week was the lessons I would learn from the patients.

I will never forget her. She was a newly diagnosed cervical cancer patient here for her first round of chemotherapy. She was only 26 years old. I walked into the infusion room where she sat in the oversized blue chair and introduced myself. Her eyes were wide open, and she sat upright with a sense of anxiety so evident on her face and in her quick movements. She smiled a small grin and told me her name. She apologized for being nervous; I told her that I, too, was nervous today because this was my first time in the clinic for an entire week, and that I was used to working during nighttime hours. I think that this eased her anxiety a little as her posture relaxed and her smile now was bigger.

After weighing her, obtaining her vital signs, and completing her education on the chemotherapy agents and the routine, I noticed that she seemed to feel much more at ease with me. She began asking me questions about my career, my southern accent (which is always a discussion topic when you are from Kentucky and living outside the area), and how I liked Tampa.

We chatted and immediately I thought to myself how much I enjoyed getting to know her. I never thought going into the week that I would be so at ease with the patients; I had all the learning expectations of skill enhancement that I would experience in the forefront of my brain. I smiled to myself with happiness, thinking this is really what it's all about.

We finished her therapy and it went well, for both of us. She tolerated the physical and mental components of her treatment with ease, and I, too, tolerated the mental components of her treatment with satisfaction, knowing that I had completed it without incident and to the best of my ability. We exchanged pleasantries, and she left. I thought about her for the next several weeks, thinking about her age and circumstance. She was so young and so brave.

A few weeks later, as I came to work, I checked my mailbox and noticed it had a card inside addressed to me here at the hospital. It was bright purple, postmarked a few days prior, and it had a huge smiley face on the back side. I was surprised to be receiving mail at work. I opened it with curiosity. Inside was a note from my special patient, thanking me for my kind and compassionate care the day she received her first round of chemotherapy.

She went on to explain how I put her at ease and how my sharing personal experiences with her kept her mind relaxed, giving her the strength to get the treatment without visible signs of sadness. You see, in the room that day, a few weeks prior, while this young woman was receiving her life-saving therapy she told me her story. She shared with me how she was diagnosed, her fears, and her plans for the future. Her greatest wish in life was to have a child, but with the course of her treatment plan, she would most likely require a hysterectomy. She hoped to adopt a child one day, but was fearful of the process. I instantly felt a special connection to this patient, and embracing that feeling, I chose to share with her a personal story of my own medical condition. I have a genetically acquired cerebral vascular malformation located in the left side of my brain, and because of the high risk of fatality with pregnancy, I, too, could not have a child. I shared with her that my husband and I hoped to adopt one day. I emphasized to her that regardless of the medical origin—whether it was cancer, infertility, or in my case, something I was born with—our paths were similar. They are not the traditional roads of motherhood. I shared with her my acceptance of this and how I believed that God had given me a different path to walk.

Little did I know the impact humanizing myself would have on my patient. That day I made a choice—rather than being the medical professional administering this toxic agent and doing only the task-oriented skills required of nursing, I chose to remove the wall of communication between patient and nurse. As I read her letter, I began to cry. I thought she was thanking me for doing my job, because being a nurse is more than learned skills—it's about helping another individual in any way possible while caring for them as a patient. My intention that day while administering her chemotherapy was to share with her my medical condition in the hope that she might not feel alone in a room associated with cancer treatment. She was in a room filled with other patients several years her senior and some of a different gender. They already had children, and some of those children were there holding the hands of the women they called "mother."

I continued to wipe the tears from my face as I read her words. I just couldn't believe it. She was the one with the fight of her life on her hands, and she took time out to thank me. I did not feel worthy. At the end of her letter, she wanted me to know that my sharing with her my personal medical history and thoughts on adoption enabled her to believe and hope for a better tomorrow. She now had accepted that her "path" was different from most, and that she would make the best of it. She did not feel alone anymore because, when she did, she thought of the "special angel with a warm smile that God had given her that day" to let her know that she was never alone.

It was during that week in the clinic that I became the patient's student, the one to learn that we might be facilitators of the health care profession, but that we are also placed in the lives of these patients for many reasons. Whatever the reason was that day, our paths crossed, and I am all the more humbled because of it. After almost 2 years in the nursing profession, I get tired and frustrated some days. However, I keep my purple card with me in my locker so that every time I open my locker, I have a reminder of why I chose nursing. When I see that card, all the frustrations that can come with being a nurse seem to disappear.

EBP Pearl

Patient preferences matter!

The Boa Constrictor That Loosened Its Grip

–Marty Adams, RN, CNIII
Eating Disorders Unit and Partial Hospitalization Program
University of North Carolina Hospitals, Chapel Hill, North Carolina

Our program opened in 2003 with a focus that is primarily cognitive-behavioral: exploring the unhealthy cognitions that lead to and maintain eating disordered behaviors and assisting patients with replacing them with healthier alternatives. The program provides an environment of structure and support to patients and their families, with a focus on assisting each patient to achieve a healthy and sustainable body weight. Our program is based on evidence-based treatments to help individuals suffering from eating disorders achieve lasting recovery. We also treat physical complications that might arise as a result of unhealthy eating or weight control practices. We are experienced in the care and treatment of comorbid psychiatric symptoms, such as anxiety and depression. Our philosophy is based on the belief that eating disorders are caused by biological, psychological, and social factors and that full recovery requires a supportive and respectful multidisciplinary approach that addresses all aspects of the individual.

On that day I first met "Mary," I was stunned to see how emaciated a person could become and still be alive. She was immobile in her bed, her muscles having wasted to unusable size and strength. She lay with her eyes closed, seemingly conserving what little energy she had. When I greeted her, she weakly responded with a soft voice and a thin smile. At this time, she was unable to do anything for herself; all of her voluntary body needs required nursing care from one or more staff, and we needed mechanical lift equipment and fabric slides as well. She presented as passive and cooperative, yet appreciative.

With mealtimes came an abrupt shift in her demeanor. She argued heatedly that we were feeding her too much. I began to realize the entrenchment of her eating disorder, thinking about how much of a challenge lay ahead for Mary and for the team.

This 34-year-old woman had suffered with anorexia nervosa since age 11 or 12 and presented to us at 42% of ideal body weight. She stayed on our eating disorders unit for only 2 hours the first time because of her medical instability. After several weeks of medical stabilization in the ICU and on the medicine unit, she came back to us for a few days until her precarious medical condition caused her to be readmitted to the medical ICU. Mary returned to us the next time for a much longer stay.

Because she was sicker than most of our eating disorders unit (EDU) patients at the time, the nursing team was concerned that we would not be able to deliver the care she needed. I had to research best practice approaches, consult with the interdisciplinary team, and stretch into some areas where I felt less confident. Mary was receiving blood transfusions, had a PICC line, an NG tube, wound care, contact precautions, and safe patient handling lift equipment. I felt a need to review how our nursing policies and procedures would have us proceed. The situation also caused me to discover changes in practices based on evidence that had occurred since the last time that I had read these documents. Armed with this data on best practices, I found that my confidence in caring for Mary's needs grew.

She was rounded on each day by the medicine service. She had daily labs drawn from a PICC line (pediatric-sized tubes to minimize the amount of blood being taken from her), and she received weekly transfusions until her own blood cell manufacturing processes were restored. The medicine team suggested that, despite her fragile medical state, the kind of psychiatric nursing care that she would receive on our unit would make the difference. This was a tremendous vote of confidence to our nursing staff, and we rose to the challenge.

Mary developed an infection and was on contact isolation for weeks. Thankfully, our nurse manager arranged for round-the-clock, one-to-one RN staffing for many days to manage the care of this very medically and psychiatrically ill woman. Repositioning was an every-2-hours affair on a special air mattress, using fabric slides, a mechanical lift, one or two nursing or OT staff, and many pillows. She was a skeleton in the bed, with thin and delicate skin stretched over bone. Edema and skin breakdown were present because of malnutrition. Expert consultation from our wound ostomy nurses, who do continuous in-house monitoring of outcomes, assisted us greatly in treating Mary's pressure wounds.

Our dietician guided the team to deliver the best nutritional approach to refeeding this patient. Initially, Mary was fed via an NG tube, which led to much "scattering" and "dropping" of food and crumbs. I created a behavior plan, "Eating Guidelines for Mary," and circulated it among my peers to gather suggestions with hopes of increasing buy-in from fellow staff. This revised document was then presented to the multidisciplinary team for their critique and support. Finally, we presented it to the patient. She was given opportunities to ask questions, challenge various points, and receive support for adhering to these guidelines. With a strong behavior plan in place, Mary progressed to feeding herself by mouth. As her self-defeating behaviors subsided, her overall condition improved, and the need for the specific plan eventually expired.

Occupational therapy (OT) contributed immensely to her regaining function. Because of a lack of muscle strength, she had been unable to lift her head. Her left arm, weaker than the right, had to be moved passively. OT worked with her daily, encouraging her, teaching her, and getting her to move her body, passively at first and then actively as she regained strength. She was retaught how to move herself, dress herself, get herself into a sitting position, and transfer to a wheelchair and then to a walker.

Physical therapy (PT) also contributed much to Mary. She was placed on their 5-day-a-week schedule. They worked with her an hour at a time and kept us informed with their evaluations of her returning strength. PT let us know what we could expect her to do for herself safely.

Mary expressed a need to have spiritual care in the form of Holy Communion and pastoral care visits. These were arranged through coordination with our Pastoral Care office and the local Catholic church.

Mary's physical recovery is nothing short of miraculous to most staff. We had such fears and concerns. I wondered if it was even possible for someone with such advanced deterioration to recover. She has surprised us all.

For weeks, she has been rolling her wheelchair around the unit. As of today, she is using a rolling walker to rebuild her ambulation skills. She no longer needs to use the wheelchair when leaving the unit for fresh-air breaks or chapel services. Her pressure ulcers are completely healed. Her previously nearly bald head is covered with new hair growth.

During the early weeks of Mary's time with us I asked her a question: "Using your imagination, what would your life be like without an eating disorder?"

She lowered her head for a minute and replied, "I want to go home."

I shared with her an idea of an image that a person with an eating disorder might be seen as being engulfed by a boa constrictor that is squeezing every bit of life out of the person. She did not respond.

Many weeks later, after she had recovered some of her strength, I revisited this question and image. To the possibility of not suffering from an eating disorder she spontaneously said, "I would have freedom, spend time with my family, have a job, and enjoy life." Her response to the boa constrictor image was, "I can tell it's getting looser and weaker."

I felt thrilled and hopeful at this improved insight. Yet, I am realistic. Mary has what is probably a lifelong chronic disease that has to be dealt with by her and her family. It could have claimed her life this year, but many professionals from many disciplines, guided by research and evidence-based practice, gave their all to achieve a very different outcome.

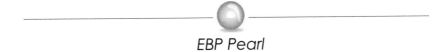

EBP Pearl

Multidisciplinary team approaches based on evidence-based practices lead to the best patient outcomes.

The UNC Eating Disorders program offers evidence-based approaches to the treatment of eating disorders, grounded on the research of Cynthia M. Bulik, PhD, the William R. and Jeanne H. Jordan Distinguished Professor of Eating Disorders in the Department of Psychiatry. Dr. Bulik is also the Professor of Nutrition in the School of Public Health and the Director of the UNC Eating Disorders Program.

Asking Questions, Finding Answers

–Natalie Carlson Drawdy, BA, RNC-MNN
Staff Nurse
Bon Secours Memorial Regional Medical Center, Mechanicsville, Virginia

It all began with a fragile young woman sitting on her bedside with her head bowed, trying to hide her tears as she looked down at the screaming baby in her arms. She was dressed modestly and wore a traditional head scarf to cover her hair. When I entered her room, she looked up at me with wide eyes that conveyed anguish and frustration so clearly it was as if she had spoken the words. Sitting down next to her, I helped her swaddle and soothe her baby. Passing her a tissue to dry her tears, I said, "Tell me about it."

I was ill-prepared for what she would tell me about a life spent in fear and turmoil, a childhood marred by gunfire and bombs, and family members who had been imprisoned, tortured, and killed. As we talked, she let me know how she had come to the United States to seek safety and stability, yet found that she was overwhelmingly lonely and isolated. At a time in her life when tradition and family were so important, she felt disconnected and alone. With only her husband for support, she felt cut off from the nurturing and care that in her culture would traditionally be provided by the women in her family. Though I didn't realize it at that moment, this experience was what launched the inquiry that led me into the world of PICO questions, quantitative and qualitative studies, and evidence-based practice.

Over the course of the next year working as a postpartum and newborn nurse, I found that I was caring for an ever-increasing number of women who were immigrants and refugees. I began asking them about their lives and what brought them to the United States. Many told me stories of growing up in places where violence and uncertainty were a way of life, of time spent in refugee camps, and of the pain of losing family and friends. The more I talked with these women and learned about their unique life stories, the more I realized the extent of the linguistic and cultural barriers they faced and how many carry significant psychological burdens with them as a result of their prior experiences. I also became convinced that this was a population that required closer screening for postpartum depression. Intuitively, I felt that by virtue of their current and past experiences, these women would harbor more predisposing risk factors for the development of the condition, and I wondered if current postpartum depression screening tools could accurately assess this very specific population.

Having begun asking the questions, I knew I needed a way to find the answers. As a nurse at the bedside, I did not consider myself a researcher, but I knew that I wanted to ensure that this special group of women was being screened adequately for postpartum depression. It was near this time that I received an e-mail calling for applications to the Clinical Scholars Program that is offered by the hospital system where I work. This program was designed to allow nurses working in clinical areas to define a problem through the development of a PICO question, teach them how to utilize and appraise research (i.e., external evidence) to find the answer, and ultimately implement evidence-based changes in clinical practice at the bedside. For 6 months, along with a small group of colleagues, I participated in monthly seminars that served as an introduction to evidence-based practice. Under the guidance of our hospital's nurse researcher, we learned how to conduct a search for the evidence, how to perform critical appraisal of studies, how to collect and analyze data, and how to develop an integrated evidence review. As a group, we shared our frustrations as we learned how to evaluate research and navigate the search for evidence. We also shared the "aha" moments as we found studies that supported evidence-based changes in clinical practice. Our nurse researcher supported us all mentally and emotionally as we made our initial forays into evidence-based practice, praising our accomplishments and helping us over the hurdles. In the end, many of us managed to take what we had discovered back to our units and use that knowledge to implement changes in patient care based on the evidence.

For my own Clinical Scholars project, and as is the case with many evidence-based projects, some answers were found and more questions were generated. I continue to search for evidence to help me understand the efficacy of postpartum depression tools when used with immigrant and refugee women. What I have learned is that I believe more research is necessary and that nurses need to strive to base their clinical practice on solid evidence. I also found the answers to some questions about myself that I didn't know I was seeking. Working with the Clinical Scholars Program led me to realize that I love research evidence and the utilization of research in implementing evidence-based practice changes in the delivery of nursing care. The program fueled my desire to take on the challenge of finding ways to answer my questions and continue my education so that I can grow in my ability as an evidence-based nurse. Ultimately, I am committed to finding the best ways of improving outcomes for immigrant women and also to inspiring my colleagues to ask questions and challenge practices to deliver the best care for our patients.

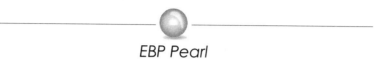

EBP Pearl

Patient preferences are central to successful EBP.

Cammy's Story

–Catherine Dukat-Wilson, RN
Psychiatric Nurse Therapist, Continuing Day Treatment Program
St. Joseph's Hospital Health Center, Syracuse, New York

Late during the evening shift at the Comprehensive Psychiatric Emergency Program (CPEP) where I worked, a young woman presented accompanied by a counselor from a local university. It was the spring of 2003, and Cammy was just 18 years old. She had been transported for an emergency psychiatric evaluation because of suicidal ideation and self-harm by cutting. Initially, nothing seemed remarkable about this troubled young woman; she was just another in a series of wounded and suffering individuals seeking some relief.

As I performed the triage process, Cammy was quiet, eyes downcast, and gave minimal responses to the questions I posed. The counselor who accompanied her was certainly more engaged in the process than the client. It was clear that Cammy wanted to be anywhere except where she was at that moment. The triage procedure completed, Cammy and her counselor were accompanied to an interview room to wait for the next steps in the process: clinical interview by a clinician, followed by a comprehensive evaluation and disposition by the attending psychiatrist.

As I went about my preparations to report off to the oncoming shift, I kept thinking about Cammy. The thoughts that replayed in my mind were, "Here is another borderline, destined to the same future as so many before her—continual hospitalizations, multiple lethal suicide attempts, and an unrelenting circle of chaos and self-harm. This can't be all that there is for her. She's just so young." I did not sleep well that night and remained troubled for many more. There just had to be something as a nurse I could do to help Cammy and others like her.

During the spring of 2006, I encountered Cammy once again, only this time as an outpatient therapist. The years since our last meeting had not been kind to Cammy. She experienced many losses, including the death of her mother, lost her role as a college student, and underwent an inpatient hospitalization at a state hospital that lasted for more than one year. For me, on the other hand, the intervening years had allowed me to be trained extensively and effectively in an evidence-based practice known as dialectical behavior therapy (DBT). Designed specifically to address the multiple needs and challenges of the client with borderline personality disorder, it provides a framework of structure and strategy to support the therapist as well. DBT became the hope I had to offer Cammy for a life that she might find worth staying alive to live. Armed with this evidence-based therapy and cautious optimism and facing my own insecurities, I began a therapeutic adventure that lasted 4 years.

Summer 2010, and implementation of this evidence-based practice in the clinical setting has transformed both me and the clients with whose care I am entrusted. The honor to participate in the healing of an individual who was initially so broken and defeated would not have been possible without DBT. Cammy has moved far beyond what many believed was probable, moved into the realm of the possible, and then moved on into reality. The growth of my own confidence and competence treating clients has exceeded my own expectations, all because of evidence, my expertise, and my patients' preferences!

As my client has changed, I have changed. She looks forward to a future of which she could not have conceived when our journey began. She is transitioning to work and back to college. I look forward to the ongoing challenge of treating those diagnosed with borderline personality disorder with an excitement and enthusiasm that was on the verge of burning out, not long ago. Evidence-based practice in nursing holds the *promise* of authentic change, the *purpose* to revolutionize patient care, and the *power* to rekindle the passion we each felt as a new nurse. Evidence-based practice brings science to the art of caring, which is the essence of nursing.

EBP Pearl

Patients matter. They are why we must practice based on evidence, and why we must be confident that EBP makes a difference!

I Will See You on the Other Side

–Nancy Robinson, BSN, RN, CCRN
Nurse Manager Emergency Department
Cincinnati VAMC, Cincinnati, OH

I have been a registered nurse for 18 years. Over the years, I have taken care of countless numbers of patients, all with their own life stories, but along the way a few special patients stand out. One patient in particular showed me the value of love, family, and faith in God. I will refer to this patient as Jim. Jim came into the emergency department initially with difficulty swallowing. I was in triage that day when we first met and was rushing through the morning trying to triage patients as quickly as I could. Jim and his wife walked in. He stood out to me because he was so tall and handsome with his dark hair and olive skin. He just had a presence about him, and his wife was equally pretty. They both stood out in a crowd together as a beautiful couple. Jim came into triage complaining of having difficulty swallowing and having food get stuck in his throat. He did not seem too concerned at the time because he had hadmultiple dilatations of an esophageal stricture in the past. Jim's vital signs were stable, and I sent him to our urgent care area for evaluation.

A few weeks later, I saw Jim and his wife walking in the hall. He smiled as he recognized me. Jim explained how he had a scope done and they found cancer. I was totally shocked. To look at Jim he was the epitome of health. How could he have cancer? I asked him a lot of questions about what they had found, but Jim had little information. He was scheduled for a biopsy in the next week. I could see great concern in both their eyes, and I had a bad feeling in my gut. I wished him luck and mentioned, "I will keep you in my prayers." He smiled and his wife thanked me; then we parted ways.

Many months went by before I saw Jim again. It was a typical busy evening shift, and I was calling patients for triage. I recognized Jim's name on the patient list, but I didn't see him in the waiting area. I called his name just to make sure, and Jim stood up. I didn't even recognize him. He was pale and gaunt, weighing 50 pounds less than the last time I saw him. His wife had changed, too. Something was very different about her face, and she looked so tired and worn. He smiled at me, and his eyes lit up and sparkled. "I am glad you are here today. You are a nice nurse," he said. He told me how he was losing his battle with esophageal cancer. The cancer had spread to the bone and the lung. He was offered hospice, but had refused. Jim explained how he was not ready to die yet and that hospice was for when you were giving up. He wasn't done fighting yet. He talked about how he was still growing his tomato plants and that he could still do things he enjoyed. He was going to live for every minute and cherish the things he loved. He talked at length about how he appreciated each day and that he talked to God more. He explained how his love for his wife and his faith in God were what had been getting him through it all. Jim seemed so positive despite his prognosis. His blood pressure was very low, and he was very ill. His body was failing, but his spirit wasn't. I took him back to the ED, and he was treated and released.

The last time I saw Jim was 2 weeks before his death. His wife came to the ED in tears. She had arrived before the ambulance. Jim's cancer had eroded into the bronchus of his lung, and he was now coughing up blood. Jim arrived minutes later. He was a shell of the man I remembered seeing a year and a half ago. He was holding a bucket full of blood and was gasping to breath. When Jim saw me, he smiled that familiar smile and had that sparkle in his eyes. He grasped my hand and then patted it. He asked me, "Are you still praying for me?" I said, "Of course I am." Jim told me he was not scared to die because he believed in Jesus. He told me about what he thought heaven would look like and that he was ready to go. Jim told me he had a good life and had no regrets except for not having more time with his wife. He seemed certain about the end of his life, and his faith was strong. I watched him struggle to breath, cough, and spatter blood. He was suffering, yet he had calmness and a sense of peace about him. It is difficult to put into words what I saw in him.

Jim wanted to die at home, spending his last hours with his family. We arranged home hospice and granted him his last request. As Jim was leaving the ED for home, he thanked me for his care and for all my prayers that helped get him through the tough times. His last words to me as he smiled with that special sparkle in his eye were, "I'll see you on the other side."

How could he be so appreciative of such simple things as a prayer or a touch in such a desperate time? I admired his faith and courage through it all. I learned a lot about myself through him. He strengthened my faith and reminded me where my focus should be in life. I look forward to seeing him again some day on the other side.

EBP Pearl

Patient preferences are essential to quality outcomes, no matter what we think about the preference or the outcome!

Making a Difference

–Lanie Welch, BSN, RN
Graduate Student
Georgia Southern University, Statesboro, Georgia

Inspiring, intense, emotional. Wow. What word truly describes the way nursing patients and making a difference in someone's life make me feel? It is amazing to me how a profession can allow me as an individual to become so connected to a complete stranger. I have been a nurse for 5 years working in the intensive care unit and as a hospice nurse. I honestly cannot put my finger on just one situation that reenergized me. It is a multitude of many patients that has changed the way I view caring for others and what remedies really work on the body, soul, and mind. I believe that it is not one story that can provide true evidence-based practice (EBP), but rather it is a long line of inspirational cases that brings the true joy of why I chose to be a nurse and the observation of how patients conquered their own sickness. These observations are part of a clinician's internal evidence used in making evidence-based decisions.

Over the years, I can remember sitting at the bedside of many patients, comforting them and speaking the truth about their condition. I can remember how holding each hand put a smile on their faces as they were unsure of what tomorrow would hold. The patients' view changed when they realized that it was not always the medicines that kept them hanging on, but the belief that they could keep living when they accepted the worst. I saw a difference in patients as they chose to take control and did not allow the worst to take control of them. I saw joy and comfort in patients as I would take the time and opportunity to listen to how they felt about their life and their condition. Listening to patients' values and preferences is an integral part of evidence-based practice.

Patients would then open up and filter out the hurt, giving themselves the opportunity to feel a sense of being. As I sat and watched the tears roll down their faces, without any words being spoken, they felt a sense of emotional relief inside: a relief to believe that medications would only allow them to prolong the natural course of life. Many of these patients came to appreciate the lives they had lived, the opportunities they had, and began to choose to appreciate the time they had left without ever looking back or feeling discouraged.

These years of experiencing this profession have allowed me to engage in the lives of many patients and has made a difference in how I view medical care. Medicine, in reality, is a choice made by a physician for treating a particular disease or illness and given to a patient that chooses to accept it. But, think about this for a moment. I ponder over all the medicines, remedies, and prescriptions that are available over a lifetime. Are these truly a sure sign of healing or just "mind over matter"? I have empathized with patients, held their hands, and comforted them when a pill could not. I have cried, laughed, and even allowed myself to be more than just their nurse. My patients learn that they can trust me. They know that I will tell them the truth even if the answers are not what they want to hear. In the end, they come to appreciate my loyalty and honesty. The patients and families choose to depend on me, and they begin to allow themselves to feel that special touch or hug that comforts instead of turning to the quick fix of what a tablet contains. It has been my prescription to nurse my patients with love, compassion, and pure quality of care; to hold their hands, allow them to feel power over their ailments, and give them a sense of dignity in coping with their conditions.

We must nurse from the heart; we must give a part of ourselves in the care we provide. We, as nurses, must take the time in providing the highest quality of care so that patients know dealing with an illness involves more than just a medicine. Patients will then come to understand that point in their illnesses when medicine stops and the soul and spirit takeover. Patients will understand that even if they don't conquer the disease, they can still prevail in the end. At that point, we must listen to their preferences and values to guide decision-making about their care.

I have experienced that some healing is from within those of us that can offer guidance, acceptance, and the willingness to be, not only a nurse, but someone that allows the feelings of our inner heart to endure, placing ourselves into the shoes of those that are depending on us to take care of them and their needs. I have seen patients and their families bond in the last days of life. I have seen patients talk to their former spouses that have gone on before them. I have seen different families choose to stop the medication, allowing nature to take its course. These families and patients are choosing to keep their loved ones comfortable, choosing to not rely on medicines to sustain life.

We all have an inner selfishness we choose to deny, but this selfishness slowly diminishes and acceptance arises, causing families to believe that the medications are no longer keeping this patient, their loved one, comfortable. The reality is often that the medicine is prolonging of a life ready to let go to move on to another place. The reality is that the medicine is causing a preventable suffering to a person whose body knows that life has made a different turn and medicine is no longer the friend, but the enemy. In witnessing this acceptance, I have seen many patients conquer their own fears, trusting in their inner faith and not what some prescription can or cannot change.

Life is a journey with many changes and choices. We have to make choices that might change life forever, but we must live through those choices. At the end of our journey, whether we choose medication, faith, or the comfort of others to relieve our pain, we all must accept patients' preferences and that the quality of lives outweighs the quantity of time. Patients turn to us for relief—relief from the hurt and sickness. Whatever the remedies used to heal or comfort, give from the heart. Nurses must have compassion that is so identifiable and assures peace for those that depend on them for comfort. We must always remember to listen to what patients want as part of evidence-based care, and always remember that the body is a vessel and does not exist without the spirit and the soul.

EBP Pearl

A patient's values and preferences must be integrated as an essential component of making evidence-based decisions.

Transcultural Nursing in Action

–Elizabeth Zicari, BSN, RN

–Louise Woerner, FAAN
HCR Home Care, Rochester, New York

Dr. Madeline Leininger, nurse theorist of transcultural nursing science, sat in our home care agency's board room. She banged her large ring on our conference table and exclaimed to our assembled nurse leaders: "Do, do, do—what is that all about?! As nurses, we need to refocus our practice away from 'do, do, do,' and take time to listen and care." By the end of that session, our leaders were all motivated and prepared to put transcultural nursing theory into practice. And what an amazing journey it has been.

One of our first acts following that encounter was to create a new team of Hispanic nurses, therapists, and home health aides who were devoted to the care of our Hispanic patients. Thanks to Dr. Leininger's work in the field of transcultural nursing, we knew we needed more to the Hispanic team than mere language skills. Any steps we could take to improve the health outcomes of our Hispanic patients would be of tremendous value, given the well-documented and significant disparities in outcomes between Hispanics and their white, non-Latino peers across the United States.

Over the years, many people in home care had come to take the poor clinical outcomes of Hispanic patients for granted, using "noncompliance" or other intractable factors as excuses for the comparative lack of success in caring for this hard-to-serve population. However, Dr. Leininger's Culture Care Theory and her Sunrise Model gave us the methodology for developing a new home care pathway for these patients; they gave us insights necessary to address and overcome those intractable factors by caring for our Hispanic patients in a culturally congruent manner.

At the core of our Hispanic team was a Puerto Rican nurse named Juanita who had a passion for improving the health of the people in her community. Juanita cared for many Hispanic home care patients, and her intuition suggested that these patients were presenting with more active diagnoses and were taking more medications than were our typical patients. As we did more research on these patients, her thoughts proved to be correct. Our Hispanic patients had an average of 7.90 active diagnoses as compared to 5.88 in our non-Hispanic patient population. Additionally, our Hispanic patients were taking an average of 14.23 medications versus 12.42 in our non-Hispanic patient population.

Mrs. Pena was one such patient. She lived in a small, one-bedroom subsidized apartment with her daughter and two very young granddaughters. Just 46, Mrs. Pena had Type 2 diabetes, blood pressure as high as 198/110, and she took several medications for her various conditions, which also included a history of anxiety and depression. She also struggled with drug and alcohol addiction, had a difficult relationship with her daughter because of the girl's own substance abuse, and was the primary caregiver for her sister who struggled with similar diagnoses.

Mrs. Pena was referred to our Hispanic home care team by a social worker at the hospital from which she had just been discharged following an admission for uncontrolled blood pressure. During that hospital stay her diabetes was first diagnosed. She had been referred to home care in the past, but hadn't accepted the service then, nor did she intend to make any changes to her diet or lifestyle after this most recent hospital stay. She was overwhelmed by this newest diagnosis of diabetes on top of all of her other issues and was becoming increasingly fatalistic with respect to her health and her prospects for improvement because of her mother's recent death from the same diseases.

When Juanita called to set up the first appointment, Mrs. Pena refused the visit. She said that she didn't want any strangers in her house. Not one to be put off easily, Juanita kept speaking patiently with her in Spanish and was eventually able to get Mrs. Pena to agree to a visit. She assured Mrs. Pena that though she might not always manage to see her herself, her care would be provided by only a few people, and they would all be Spanish-speaking.

Juanita and others on the Hispanic team had been using Leininger's Sunrise Model to capture insights into our Hispanic patients' educational and economic factors, cultural values, beliefs, and lifeways, and to understand and appreciate patients' environmental context, such as language and ethnohistory. A new care pathway that took these into account and that leveraged, rather than ignored, Hispanic cultural nuances that had emerged was refined by the team over time.

At that first home visit with Mrs. Pena, Juanita took Dr. Leininger's advice to heart and started the visit by listening rather than doing. Mrs. Pena said, "I am really tired of being ill." She talked about her mother's death 2 years earlier and how much she missed her. Mrs. Pena eventually revealed that she was illiterate and could only write her name and recognize numbers. She described her resentment that she was treated as stupid by the health care system, which helped to explain why she had refused home care in the past. Juanita learned that Mrs. Pena didn't understand her medications, nor could she afford them. Through listening to Mrs. Pena and taking into consideration her values and preferences as part of delivering evidence-based care, a new understanding of Mrs. Pena's and many other Hispanic patients' histories of "noncompliance" began to emerge. A social worker on the Hispanic team managed to put together the resources needed so Mrs. Pena could obtain her medications. The challenge then became how to provide the education and motivation necessary for her to take them consistently and correctly.

Using Mrs. Pena's mother's early death and her fierce love of her granddaughters as a motivator, Juanita set a goal of educating her about one medication on each visit. Mrs. Pena had consistently refused to take one of her medications, and ultimately, Juanita determined that she was afraid to take it because of her drinking. Juanita encouraged Mrs. Pena by using the strengths-based approach that is a cornerstone of transcultural nursing practice, showing her how her discipline in the care of her sister could be similarly applied to stopping her use of drugs and alcohol. When Mrs. Pena still refused to take the medication, Juanita told her, "Go ahead and die and leave your grandchildren, just like your mother left you." After a pause, Mrs. Pena replied that no one had ever said that to her before, and she agreed to try to stop the alcohol and drug use that had been dragging her down for so long. From that point forward, Juanita and Mrs. Pena were in a different relationship; trust now existed because Juanita had applied aspects of the Sunrise Model (and tough love) to her approach.

In the weeks to come, Juanita even began diabetic teaching, thanks to Mrs. Pena's new receptivity. However, given the literacy challenges in this case, the use of mainstream diabetic meal plans and cookbooks wasn't an option. Furthermore, Juanita and the rest of the Hispanic team had found that they often had greater success when advocating portion control for their diabetic patients, rather than trying to replace culturally important foods such as rice and beans with unfamiliar foods. In Mrs. Pena's case, Juanita made use of the Idaho Plate Method to teach portion control and the appropriate ratios for protein, fruits and vegetables, starches, and dairy products.

Together Mrs. Pena and Juanita reviewed the steps by which Mrs. Pena would check her blood sugar and what to do given various readings. Juanita also focused on reducing the salt in Mrs. Pena's diet. After preparing one such meal, Mrs. Pena said to Juanita in a tone of surprise, "It didn't taste that bad!"

Mrs. Pena's very low level of literacy was a challenge in medication management as well. Her Mediset was marked with times of day, but she couldn't read them. Juanita removed the boxes from the Mediset that weren't needed by Mrs. Pena, leaving just one for morning and one for evening each day. Then she helped Mrs. Pena to learn a system by which she could use a box's color to remind her when those pills should be taken: blue like the sky in the morning and red like the setting sun in the evening.

Mrs. Pena responded well. She felt empowered by the teaching, and learned her medications. She realized that she didn't have to die young from a stroke resulting from high blood pressure. Between modifications to her diet and consistent use of her medications, she could live a long life. She stopped using drugs and alcohol. She could live to enjoy her daughter and her grandchildren, as she had hoped her mother would. After a month's time she was discharged from our agency's care, with a controlled blood pressure of 120/70 and a newfound confidence that stemmed from having trust in our nurse.

On the day of her final nursing visit, Mrs. Pena asked Juanita if she could still talk with her when she saw her in the building. Juanita looked at her fondly and answered, "I'll always be your nurse."

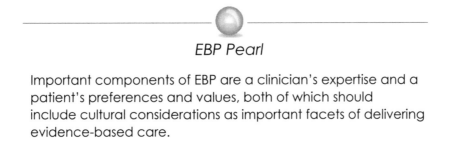

EBP Pearl

Important components of EBP are a clinician's expertise and a patient's preferences and values, both of which should include cultural considerations as important facets of delivering evidence-based care.

4

Improving Outcomes With Evidence-Based Practice

A paradigm can be viewed as how you think about something. The evidence-based (EBP) practice paradigm is about integrating valid (i.e., well done) research with clinicians' expertise (e.g., skills in assessing patients, resource utilization, and the EBP process) and preferences and values of patients for the purpose of improving outcomes. Without a focus on outcomes, the EBP paradigm and process become meaningless. Outcomes have been on the forefront of such quality initiatives as the Institute for Healthcare Improvement (IHI) and the Centers for Medicaid and Medicare Services (CMS). Increasingly, care providers have outcome data to reflect their impact on care. The stories in this chapter reflect how clinicians have approached decision-making from the evidence-based practice paradigm and process perspective to make a wonderful positive difference in patient, provider, and system outcomes...enjoy!

The Visible Power of Nurses Doing the Right Thing Right: "Say Aaahhh!"

–*Cecelia L. Crawford, MSN, RN*
Kaiser Permanente Southern California, Patient Care Services, Regional Nursing Research Program
Kaiser Permanente, Southern California, Pasadena, California

–*Lynne M. Scott, MN, RN, CCRN, CCNS*
Department Administrator, Dialysis, Clinical Nurse Specialist Critical Care and DOU
Kaiser Foundation Hospitals, Woodland Hills, Woodland Hills, California

It started with a nurse's question of "What is the best way to care for a patient's mouth?" The answer to that mundane question ended up driving the activities of a 13-member Kaiser Permanente (KP) Nursing Practice Council (NPC) for 3 years. These activities required partnerships with KP nursing leadership, materials management, and pharmacy, as well as consultation with a dentist and collaboration with a national oral care products company. When the journey ended, the nurses not only improved a medical center's structure and processes surrounding the care of the patient's mouth, but also caused a systems change in the way KP Southern California itself practices oral health. Along the way, the NPC learned how to make the invisible work of nurses visible and how important it was to do the right thing right.

Many nurses consider oral care a distasteful, but basic nursing activity. This low-tech activity is often underestimated in a high-tech nursing environment. The KP Woodland Hills NPC decided to tackle this patient care task as an evidence-based practice (EBP) project, as the issue of oral care cut across the units represented by its members. We selected the Iowa Model of Evidence-Based Practice to Promote Quality Care as the EBP project's framework to investigate the evidence and implement a consistent oral care protocol for the compromised hospitalized patient. In addition to providing nurses with a structure to transform their nursing practice, the Iowa Model also highlighted the organizational needs of Kaiser Permanente. At first, the staff nurses found the model complex and intimidating. However, they soon found that they could easily navigate the model's simple algorithmic nature. Within a few months, empowered NPC members were verbally outlining and explaining the systematic processes necessary for an EBP project to be successful and sustainable. As a group, we decided to use an open mouth as the project's branded visible logo, later re-enforced by the title of "Say Aaahhh!"

The "Say Aaahhh!" identifying image assists nurses in choosing specific products to individualize a patient's oral care and provides a visual aid for the restocking of supplies. The NPC conducted an exhaustive review of the evidence surrounding oral care practices in the acute care setting. It became clear that the invisible work by nurses was exemplified by the practice of oral care. The literature was replete with information on the value of oral care for patients who were intubated or receiving chemotherapy and about the link between oral care and ventilator-associated pneumonia. However, very little evidence existed for other types of compromised hospitalized patients. The initial evidence search allowed the NPC to streamline the project's focus to three distinct patient populations: the frail elderly patient, the ventilated ICU patient, and the adult or pediatric patient receiving chemotherapy. One phrase that struck a chord with NPC members concerned frail elderly patients needing oral care, who were described as being "neglected and disenfranchised." These three words raised our consciousness and renewed our determination to do the right thing right by developing an oral care protocol for the compromised patient.

With new vigor, the NPC crafted evidence-based recommendations that eventually populated the "Say Aaahhh!" oral care protocol and preprinted orders specifically designed for these at-risk hospitalized patients. A few short sentences summed up the protocol and became our mantra: "Brush to clean, followed by chlorhexidine, swab in-between." During the protocol design, the NPC members made the groundbreaking decision to include the antimicrobial agent chlorhexidine (CHG) as a swish-and-spit or swabbed application. Although the research evidence was weak, the Iowa Model led trailblazing staff nurses through the decision-making process of examining the risks versus the benefits of CHG and to consulting with a dental expert. After reviewing the research evidence and discussing the proposed protocol, the dentist consultant convinced us that the benefits of decreased microbial activity in the mouth outweighed the risks of discolored teeth, which is easily resolved with one teeth-cleaning visit. NPC members had to convince many physicians, nurses, pharmacists, and other health care professionals of CHG's value for this new protocol to be accepted. In May 2010, the Institute for Healthcare Improvement added the element of routine CHG use in their ventilator bundle update, which reaffirms that we made the right decision as based on the best evidence available.

What was the current state of the patient's mouth? Two NPC nurses volunteered to lead the preintervention oral assessment and documentation review on select pilot units to determine current oral care practices. These same nurses enthusiastically conducted the postintervention oral assessment and documentation review on the pilot units to evaluate the effectiveness of the intervention. The postevaluation results and staff nurse feedback led to modifications of the protocol and order sets as per the Iowa Model. The NPC then took charge of expanding the oral care protocol throughout the remainder of the hospital's acute care units, with monthly snapshot audits of oral assessment and documentation over a 3-month period. Although these activities sound simple to implement and monitor, the actual time and effort involved was considerable. However, the NPC nurses' passion kept the EBP project alive and visible.

While the pilot was taking place, other NPC nurses evaluated the oral care products being used and determined that they were not aligned with the evidence. In a bold move, the nurses contacted a national oral care products company and asked if a small batch of unique products could be designed that met the evidence recommendations. To our surprise and delight, the company flew their marketing director and support sales staff from Chicago to California to meet with select NPC members. Our dialogue resulted in oral care products that were not only based on the evidence, but were also designed by nurses who use them and who are familiar with the patients who need them. This meeting was the beginning of a 2-year partnership that not only developed oral care items specific to "Say Aaahhh!" but also led the company to eventually develop existing oral care product lines and recommendations that in essence mirror our home-grown EBP project. This partnership experience was an epiphany regarding the power of nurses and taking advantage of being in the right place at the right time.

Three KP EBP grants supported the protocol design, consultation fees, and the staff nurse-driven pilot project activities for the first year, and continued with data collection and data entry during the second year. The third EBP grant allowed the NPC the new experience of hiring an outside statistician to "crunch the numbers." Did the "Say Aaah-hh!" oral care protocol make a difference for the compromised hospitalized patient? The answer was conflicting because our pilot sample was too small to reach statistical signifi-cance for some outcomes. Although intubated patients received more per-shift average oral care than nonintubated patients, no other significant differences existed between patient subgroups, nor was there a significant relationship between the oral assessment scores and how long a patient was intubated. There were no significant differences in oral assessment scores among the different patient populations. However, there were observable trends reflecting improved oral assessment scores and frequency of per-shift oral care—both good results! This was when we learned that, though the results were not statistically significant, they were definitely clinically significant. The data also vali-dated the research evidence regarding missed opportunities for at-risk patients to receive oral care, particularly for frail elderly patients.

The NPC nurses reviewed the data results, discussed the clinical implications, re-solved not to give up, and pledged to continue to do the right thing. The NPC chair herself led a yearlong campaign to have the protocol converted to an electronic order set and successfully navigated the bureaucratic channels to assure its inclusion in Health-Connect, KP's electronic health care record. NPC members negotiated with the na-tional oral care products company to continue to manufacture the oral care products and have them available for KP medical centers wanting to use the "Say Aaahhh!" protocol. Those two activities enable any KP facility in the nation to institute an evidence-based oral care protocol for their own unique compromised hospitalized patient populations.

The invisible work of KP nursing has been made visible not only by improving pa-tient documentation, oral assessment, and data analysis, but also through the NPC staff nurses' dissemination of information via various presentations and information given to key organizational groups. These activities capture the Iowa Model's emphasis on widespread information dissemination. Many NPC members still cannot believe they not only changed one medical center's oral care practices, but also spread this practice change throughout the KP California region and impacted a national health care organiza-tional system. By doing the right thing right, the NPC staff nurses have improved the oral care of compromised hospitalized frail elderly patients, intubated patients, and adult and pediatric oncology patients with an evidence-based demonstration of high quality patient care. What is the best way to care for a patient's mouth? "Say Aaahhh!"

EBP Pearl

Evidence-based practice is doing the right thing to improve quality of care and patient outcomes!

"Take Two: My Finale"

–Élise Arsenault Knudsen, MS, RN
Evidence-Based Practice Clinical Nurse Specialist
University of Wisconsin Hospital and Clinics, Madison, Wisconsin

Rarely in life do we get the opportunity for a "do-over," and it essentially never happens in the life of a bedside nurse. However, we can experience the uplifting feeling of success when we "live and learn," and from that learning, we can make a difference in the lives of the patients that we touch.

During my routine shift on that rainy spring day, I wasn't thinking about all the patients that had influenced my care over the last 7 years of my tenure as a bedside nurse; my focus was solely on the four patients for whom I had to care, two of whom needed to be discharged, and the one who was still to come up from the ICU later that day. When I received report from the ICU on "my patient," I didn't know that he was going to be one of the last patients I would care for as a staff nurse or the effect that he and his family would have on me. Or even how, months later, I would be able to look back on the care I provided for him and his family as some of the best care I ever gave a patient, attributable to the hundreds of patients I had cared for before him, the knowledge I had accumulated, and the support of an amazing staff.

The unit-to-unit report began as usual—name, age, attending physician, admission date, and diagnosis. It wasn't until the list of injuries were being described to me over the phone that it happened; I had a feeling (you know that feeling) that I was going to have a chance to do this right, I mean really right. The litany of injuries this patient endured from his motorcycle crash was eerily similar to ones that another patient I had cared for had suffered 3 years prior. Furthermore, the same room on the unit that previous patient had stayed in had just opened up, and this new patient was to be placed there. It was easy for me to flash back to the patient I had cared for 3 years earlier, remembering the rollercoaster ride of his hospitalization and the stress it caused the nursing staff. Trying to focus on this patient instead of recalling my past patient, I finished receiving the report, hung up the phone, and said to myself, "Here we go again."

What amazed me was how over the next few weeks this patient, who should have been extraordinarily complex to care for, was instead like doing a repeat performance, but even easier. I knew from past experiences, from the support of the interdisciplinary staff, and from the literature that I had read how to mold his plan of care to improve his outcomes. As his sensation in his lower extremities returned and the pain increased, I drew on this knowledge to advocate for improved pain control. As I attempted to bend over my ever-growing pregnant belly to pack his multiple wounds several times a shift, I assessed the copious drainage and odor from them, and I knew that, unfortunately, those wounds had more to their stories—and they did. As I patiently stood or sat at the patient's bedside and listened to the concerns of the patient and the family, I could offer reassurance because I knew in my gut that he would be okay; though what "okay" meant was yet to be determined. In discussing his plan of care, I could speak confidently with the team, take into consideration his whole self, and not just focus on the infections, his antibiotics, nausea, pain, and next OR date.

With the help of the entire nursing staff and his family, we developed a plan of care to maximize his health and to avoid the preventable. Three years before his admission to our unit, we had undertaken an evidence-based practice (EBP) project to help increase awareness of patients at risk for pressure ulcers and to decrease the incidence of pressure ulcers on the unit. Heeding the suggested interventions outlined in our project, I entered his room every 2 hours to assure that we turned and repositioned him, ensuring comfort and shifting his body weight. As I encouraged his participating in therapy and drinking protein shakes, and as I completed my daily head-to-toe skin assessment, I knew that I was providing the best care. When a spot on the back of his head started to lose hair from the pressure of being bedridden for many weeks, I knew enough to not hesitate in his treatment and, therefore, prevented breakdown. When I lamented to our Wound and Skin Clinical Nurse Specialist over the smaller-than-a-pencil-eraser pressure spot on his Achilles, she assured me I was doing everything possible to facilitate healing and that indeed I should be applauded for only one worry spot after the patient had been hospitalized and in bed for 47 days.

When the patient was beginning to show signs of hopelessness and simply wanted to get out of his room, my coworkers and I wheeled him out of his room into the hallway in his bed with full trapeze intact so that he could see other people walk by and hear different sounds. I discovered a basic realization by witnessing the smile on his face—this is truly what it means to be a nurse.

Evidence-based practice is the conscientious use of best evidence coupled with clinician experience and patient's values. More nurses are talking about how practice rooted in evidence will lead to improved patient outcomes. What isn't part of that definition is the sense of satisfaction the nursing staff feels when they know they have provided the best care they know how to do. What isn't included in that definition is how improved patient outcomes are translated on the face of the patient, his wife, or his mother when they say "thank you" and give you a hug. What isn't included in that definition is the trusting relationship that is developed for patients to say "yes" to a new drug, a new dressing, a new therapy, or another trip to the OR because the patient knows that their input is being weighed as part of the equation.

In those final weeks of my life as a bedside nurse, I cared for this patient day after day as his primary nurse, applying to his care the knowledge and skills that I had learned from everything I had done over the previous 7 years. When I said goodbye to him and his family as I had so many other shifts before, I didn't know it was going to be my last.

And when just a few days later I crossed the stage to receive my master's degree in nursing, and then days after that delivered my second child, I knew that my life as a bedside nurse was over. But more importantly, I knew that I had done my job and had done it well.

Today, new to my role as a Clinical Nurse Specialist for EBP, I am once again inspired and awed at the impact nurses have in the lives of our patients (not to mention the reverse). As I make my transition from a staff nurse to a Clinical Nurse Specialist, my goal is to support my nurse colleagues' spirit of inquiry and the continual quest for providing evidence-based nursing care and, in turn, to allow others to feel a great sense of achievement and satisfaction by knowing they are providing the best care possible.

EBP Pearl

Evidence-based practice not only leads to the highest quality of care and improves patient outcomes, but also enhances job satisfaction and fulfillment in clinicians.

Surviving Sepsis Campaign—How One Nurse Became a Believer

–Lori E. Geisler, MSN, RN, CCRN
Clinical Nurse Specialist, Critical Care
Shore Health System, Easton, Maryland

In 2008, our hospitals implemented an evidence-based sepsis bundle to reduce the mortality rate of patients with severe sepsis. One example of how well these evidence-based interventions can work involves a young male septic patient in our intensive care unit (ICU) who was severely hypotensive and without urine output, despite many liters of IV fluids. He, in fact, appeared to be fluid overloaded. Our sepsis protocol called for me to check central venous oxygen saturations ($ScvO_2$) on the patient every 2 hours. The initial saturation was in normal range. Given that our ICU had recently purchased continuous $ScvO_2$ monitors and catheters and that a central line needed to be placed to measure central venous pressure (CVP), the attending physician and I decided to place an oxymetric central catheter, thereby facilitating both CVP and $ScvO_2$ monitoring on a continuous rather than intermittent basis. Our clinical expertise helped us to most efficiently use the health care resources we had available.

After the line was placed, we found the CVP to be very high, and the attending physician and intensivist consulted a nephrologist who decided that this patient needed to be dialyzed for fluid overload, hyperkalemia, and metabolic acidosis. The surgeon was called to place the dialysis catheter. While awaiting the surgeon's arrival, I noticed that the $ScvO_2$ was dropping, indicating, by our evidence-based protocol, that I needed to start a Dobutamine infusion. Within 15 minutes of my initiating the Dobutamine, the patient began making urine. The nephrologist, intensivist, and attending physician agreed to hold off on the dialysis catheter for a little while. The patient's $ScvO_2$, BP, and urine output all improved, with lab work improving within a few hours. Two days later the patient was extubated and had normal chemistries without ever receiving dialysis or even having a dialysis access placed. He was discharged from ICU the day after extubation and discharged from the hospital 2 days after that.

If we had not placed the oximetric central line, 2 hours would have passed before the drop in $ScvO_2$ was recognized. The patient would have received his dialysis catheter and had hemodialysis initiated within that timeframe. Continuous $ScvO_2$ monitoring saved this patient from unnecessary procedures, reduced his length of time in the ICU and hospital, and perhaps saved his life.

This day taught me the true value of each intervention we perform. Following our evidence-based protocols really does improve patient outcomes.

EBP Pearl

Evidence-based protocols, when blended with clinical expertise, save lives!

A Nurse's Impact on Better Patient Outcomes: Formation of a Support Group

–*Lucy Artinian, MN, RN, FNP*
Lecturer
UCLA School of Nursing, Los Angeles, California

After I graduated with a master's degree in nursing, I was offered a position as a Clinical Nurse Specialist (CNS) at a major university-affiliated gastroenterology (GI) group. This outpatient practice with a clinical and research focus included several physicians, fellows, and residents specialized in inflammatory bowel disease (IBD), namely Crohn's disease and ulcerative colitis. I was excited with this new direction in my nursing career where I could further my knowledge of GI diseases and hopefully have a direct positive impact on patient care.

As a Clinical Nurse Specialist/Nurse Coordinator, I greeted all patients who came to the clinic and spent time with them before and after a physician met with them. I then provided the patients with information about their diseases and discussed their medications and upcoming tests, the need for referrals to other specialists, and occasionally, the possible need for surgery. I responded to their daily calls, inquired about their symptoms, allayed their concerns, tapered medications per the physicians' guidelines, and reassured them that disease remission was our main treatment goal. Occasionally, when they experienced severe flare-ups of their symptoms and needed hospitalization, I visited them daily and brought their needs and concerns to both the nursing and medical teams. In summary, I was their advocate within the confines of a large university hospital system and made every effort to contribute to their personalized medical care when they were admitted.

Numerous daily responsibilities kept me very busy; however, I greatly enjoyed my interactions with the patients and the ability to assist them through the many stages of their illnesses. As an intermediary between the patients and the physicians, I became a trusted confidante for my patients; I knew them, and they counted on me to bring their needs to the physician's attention. However, I soon realized that I mostly followed "doctors' orders" and relayed back their instructions to the patients. As a new graduate with an advanced nursing degree, I was consumed with ideals that I had gathered in school. I was eager to intervene directly and have a greater impact on my patients' ability to cope with a chronic ailment.

After several months of work, I became acutely aware and greatly familiar with the many needs of this patient population. Patients with IBD are mostly young adults in their 20s and 30s. The severity of their symptoms (severe abdominal pain and cramping due to bowel obstruction in Crohn's disease, and severe bloody diarrhea with up to 10 bowel movements a day in ulcerative colitis) often takes a toll on them, their families, and their quality of life.

The inspiration to form a support group for patients with IBD developed gradually over several months. The many needs of our young adult patients compelled me to help them improve their coping skills. In doing so, I would directly contribute to their ability to manage their symptoms and improve their daily lives. I was confident that "patient-to-patient support" would serve as an adjunct to the services provided by our professional group practice and mark a positive contribution by me as its CNS.

Patient-to-patient support groups are based on the premise that support from other individuals with a similar experience can help reduce the negative impact of the disease and improve the ability to cope. Findings from several studies document the positive effects of support groups, and a literature search revealed the following evidence: Support groups enhance patients' self-esteem, self-efficacy, and confidence and provide social support and spiritual well-being. In addition, participation in support groups is associated with significant improvement in patients' emotional state, illness adaptation, quality of life, and marital relationships.

In graduate school, our professors ingrained in us the concept that nurses are in an ideal position to positively impact patient outcomes. Therefore, the formation of a support group seemed a tremendous opportunity to implement evidence-based practice (EBP) and to document nurses' contributions to positive patient outcomes. The physicians I worked with were extremely supportive and encouraged me to initiate my plan to form a patient support group. Also, they were eager to learn whether the support group would make a significant contribution to their patients' general well-being.

Although I had the willingness, the certitude, and the determination to begin a patient support group, I recognized that I needed leadership assistance from peers in graduate school with a specialty in psychiatric nursing. My peers were better prepared to interact and enhance therapeutic communications between patients. Two nurses volunteered to lead the group and, thus, began a collaboration that lasted 10 years and helped hundreds of patients with IBD.

The IBD Support Group met regularly, once a month, for one and a half hours. Eight to ten patients attended each session. I organized the group, sent reminder letters, called patients a few days before the meeting, and passed out flyers in clinic. I reserved the room, brought in refreshments, and occasionally, scheduled physicians and nurses to serve as guest lecturers for the group. However, the patients led most of the discussions. They shared their concerns, their struggles, and their triumphs over the negative effects of the disease. After each session, we found great encouragement to discover new friendships formed and personal information exchanged between patients in the group. Older patients shared their stories and tips with younger ones, and the younger patients energized all the participants with their liveliness and "can do" attitude. The mutual support and care for each individual's struggle was evident at each session. The group leaders directed the discussion and encouraged everyone to participate. I contributed to the discussions when discrepancies in medical information came up or when clarification was important. We, the leaders, came to know each patient well. They, in turn, developed a trusting relationship with us.

Just as research continues to document the positive impact of support groups on patient outcomes, we also observed this to be the case in our group of patients. Over the years, we observed mutual care and support amongst the participants. They engaged in one another's struggles, discussed information about insurance plans and their concerns for inadequate health coverage, and shared knowledge of new medications and alternative therapies. Over time, social bonds formed, and new relationships burgeoned. Often, patients described how appreciative they were to participate and find safety in a group of people afflicted with a similar condition. We, the group leaders, also noted that patients who attended the group regularly were better able to cope with their disease. The patients were better informed about their illness and its long-term consequences; they came to their appointments regularly, took their medications as prescribed, inquired about alternatives therapies, and requested these in addition to standard treatment. They were more assertive and actively participated in their plan of care. Consequently, our support group did indeed contribute and enhance each patient's day-to-day ability to cope with their disease. Over time, these abilities could reduce their stress level and improve their quality of life. An encouraging testament to the positive impact of our support group is the fact that it has lasted for 10 years, thus validating its relevance to and its immense value for people who face a chronic, long-term disease like IBD.

Over the years, this IBD Support Group became a most cohesive group of patients and, eventually, friends. Although some patients came only a few times a year, the core group members were often present and leading the discussions. As the support group became known within the community, we received many referrals from other gastroenterology centers throughout the community.

I was the CNS for the IBD outpatient clinic for 9 years; however, the support group continued even after I left. Sometimes, I remember I was reluctant to attend the meetings after a long day of work. That reluctance quickly faded into an immense energy during the meeting, and I was stirred by positive emotions after I left every meeting. On the way home, I often replayed in my head all the stimulating interactions that took place that evening and how greatly patients benefit from the input of others with intimate knowledge of their personal experience.

I consider the initiation and organization of the IBD Support Group and its steady 10-year survival as one of the proudest achievements of my nursing career. I always knew nurses could have a direct impact on quality care and apply EBP within their work setting to improve patient outcomes: our IBD Support Group made this a reality.

EBP Pearl

Taking the initiative to implement practices based on the best evidence from research improves patients' outcomes and lives.

Implementation of a Bedside Swallowing Tool

–*Rhonda Babine, MS, RN, ACNS-BC*
Adult Health Clinical Nurse Specialist, Geriatrics
Maine Medical Center, Portland, Maine

–*Anne-Marie Hardman, MSN, RN, ACNS-BC, OCN, CIC*
Adult Health Clinical Nurse Specialist, Oncology
Southern Maine Medical Center, Biddeford, Maine

In January of 2008, Rhonda began her first semester of clinical experience in the adult health clinical nurse specialist program at the University of Southern Maine. The facility, Southern Maine Medical Center, is a 150-bed hospital within the Maine Health System. One expectation of the clinical experience for the clinical nurse specialist student is to complete a clinical project that will advance the practice of nursing at the institution. In the state of Maine, prior to June of 2008, a nurse performing swallowing assessments on patients at risk for aspiration was not considered within the scope of practice of the registered nurse (RN). Rhonda and Anne-Marie discussed the needs of acute stroke patients and the need for more education for nursing staff. These conversations led them down a road where the care of patients experiencing a stroke at Southern Maine Medical Center would be forever changed.

Dysphagia has been reported to occur in about half of all acute stroke patients. One of the stroke performance measurements for accreditation by the Joint Commission includes a screen for dysphagia on all ischemic/hemorrhagic stroke and transient ischemic attack (TIA) patients before being given food, fluids, or medication by mouth. In a small community hospital, a speech pathologist is not always available to perform swallowing evaluations. Furthermore, the majority of the patients evaluated by a speech pathologist have negative assessments. The delay in assessment was concerning to us because, depending on the day and time of admission, patients might remain without oral intake and oral medications from several hours to days, leading to a decrease in patient satisfaction and possibly a risk of aspiration when the patient drinks or eats during this time. Because of the high volume of patients that must be evaluated by a speech pathologist, more critical patients might not receive needed care in a timely manner. Health care dollars also are lost with the charge of a potentially unnecessary formal swallowing evaluation by a speech pathologist. If nursing could do an initial assessment to screen patients so that the low-risk patients could eat and drink and the high-risk patients could be referred to a speech pathologist for further evaluation, overall patient care would be improved.

We performed a literature search and found that the practice of the RN performing bedside swallowing screens is evidence-based. However, at Southern Maine Medical Center, the skill was not included in the competency of the RN, and it was not listed in the scope of practice for the RN with the State Board of Nursing. To improve the patient care of this population, we knew the practice of RNs performing bedside swallowing assessments needed to be added to the scope of practice in the state of Maine.

After several conversations with the speech pathologist in the hospital, we again turned to the evidence by searching the literature, looking to find an evidenced-based bedside swallowing tool that could be administered by an RN. The Toronto Bedside Swallowing Screening Test (TOR-BSST) is an algorithm for performing bedside swallowing screens by professionals other than speech pathologists. Studies have demonstrated a 19% increase in appropriate speech referrals with the utilization of this tool. One determent to implementing this tool into practice is that the buy-in from the speech pathologist is imperative because the skill must be taught by a licensed speech pathologist.

Before we could begin educating nurses in using the tool, we had to inquire with the State Board of Nursing regarding the scope of practice. Anne-Marie was in contact with the Board of Nursing regarding the process to add the skill to the scope of practice for the RN in the state of Maine. A survey for addressing questions regarding nursing practice was completed and sent to the State Board of Nursing for review. The State Board of Nursing representative made the decision to present the questionnaire and the practice question to the board in June, which was 3 months away. Unfortunately, we did not want to wait that long for implementation. The data we reviewed spoke volumes to us; it was not good practice to make a patient wait for a swallowing assessment to be completed, especially when in most states and hospitals, including Maine, swallowing assessments performed by RNs were commonplace, utilizing homegrown tools not based on evidence and patient outcomes.

To begin a pilot program utilizing a new skill prior to the Maine State Board of Nursing approval, we were required to complete a Scope of Practice Decision Tree. The Scope of Practice Decision Tree required the approval of the chief nursing officer (CNO) at Southern Maine Medical Center. We met with the CNO and presented the evidence from the literature search, supporting data, and the projected project plan of implementation. To ensure patient safety, the CNO recommended we proceed with a pilot program beginning with nursing education and implementation of the swallowing tool in May of 2008.

To make certain that nursing education was complete, we implemented an assessment of the nursing knowledge in the basic pathophysiology and care of the stroke patient. Our assessment concluded that 50% of nurses at Southern Maine Medical Center considered a swallowing deficit on all patients admitted with a stroke. Nurses stated that 75% of the time they would initiate a speech pathologist referral only if a swallowing difficulty was noted. All nurses stated that if they had a question of a swallowing difficulty they would attempt giving the patient water. Nurses would then subjectively make a decision on whether the patient was safe with swallowing. The nurses used no objective tool to assess this, and they had an evident deficit in knowledge in the care of the stroke patient. The educational plan was based on our assessments of the nursing learning needs identified with surveys and observation. In collaboration with speech pathology, we developed an educational offering that included stroke education, aspiration/swallowing education, TOR-BSST tool for bedside swallowing screening, and a return demonstration/simulation of TOR-BSST tool for bedside swallowing screening. At the end of the educational offering, nurses completed a competency verification tool. It is important to note that TOR-BSST education must be provided by a licensed speech pathologist. To begin the project as a pilot, we selected a small group of nurses on a medical telemetry unit to complete the education including both the nursing unit manager and the unit coordinator.

One consideration for the completion of this initiative included developing the TOR-BSST screen within the electronic documentation system. The nursing informatics specialist provided invaluable assistance. The assessment includes the three following questions that evaluate a patient's swallowing status:

1. Do you have dysphagia or difficulty swallowing?

2. Is there a depressed cough or gag reflex present?

3. Have you had a recent stroke/TIA?

A positive response to any of the three questions indicates that the RN will complete the TOR-BSST form and place it in the patient's medical record. The swallowing screening procedure indicating the patient has passed the screen consists of the patient swallowing 10 sips of water without coughing or garbled speech. The patient who fails the TOR-BSST screen is restricted on oral intake, including oral medications, until the speech therapist can evaluate the patient further. The RN notifies the physician of the restricted oral intake status and obtains an order for medications to be held or given parenterally. The patient who passes the TOR-BSST screen does not have any changes in diet or medication administration.

Another consideration for the completion of this initiative included the development of a policy and procedure for the swallowing assessment by the RN. Also, we engaged the physicians in the program by educating them on the validity and reliability of the TOR-BSST swallowing screen.

In June of 2008, as a result of our project, the Maine Board of Nursing determined that it is within the scope of practice of the RN to conduct a swallow assessment after completion of education and verification of competency. We have had this assessment in place since May of 2008. The speech pathologist, Arlene Baker MS, CCC-SLP, MSM, has documented that swallowing evaluation orders are appropriate 93% of the time. Patients are restricted on oral intake only when necessary, and the physicians have supported the validity of the tool. Two years later, it is evident that with the implementation of a bedside swallowing tool that is evidence-based, patient care and patient satisfaction have been improved at Southern Maine Medical Center.

EBP Pearl

Students working together with staff who have a spirit of inquiry along with persistence to implement the steps of evidence-based practice can transform care and improve outcomes for vulnerable patients.

Enhancing the Recovery of a Stroke Survivor: Bridging the Gap in the Community

–Christina Ball, RN, CNRN
Shore Health System, University of Maryland Medical System
Easton, Maryland

For 10 very short years, I have been a neuroscience nurse. In my most recent experience, I have had the fortunate opportunity of coordinating my community hospital's stroke center. I have always loved caring for stroke patients, and before I became the stroke center coordinator, I really thought the care I delivered in the hospital was the most valuable part of their recovery. Located in a rural setting where resources are limited, our hospital plays a major role in ensuring that our community receives the health services that they require. Little did I know that my eyes were about to be opened to a world that I had overlooked.

The story really begins when I received a phone call from a stroke survivor in the community, inquiring about the availability of a stroke support group. Developing the support group had been on my to-do list, but our conversation led to the development of something amazing: the Talbot County Stroke Support Group. Today, that group consists of 35 members and is growing every day. We have shared tears, laughter, and successes and have developed relationships that have impacted our lives forever. It has allowed me to see the world of stroke survivors through their eyes and has given a new meaning to the word "survivor."

The physical and psychological effects of stroke can often transform one's environment into a threatening one. Over time, I began to realize that we could enhance the care we were delivering to stroke patients while they are in the hospital. From the stroke survivors, I learned what emotions they felt, their struggles, the rehabilitation opportunities that were never given to them, their insurance nightmares, and the things that they had wished they were told in the hospital. I began to recognize that the focus of caring for a patient with a stroke needed to include developing a discharge plan that would maximize their recovery in various dimensions. The period following discharge has been described as the most challenging for stroke survivors. By using a team approach, we began to put the pieces in place for patients to optimize their recovery from their stroke and bridge the gap back into the community, thereby defragmenting their care.

Incorporating an assessment for rehabilitation services is one of the most important aspects of the stroke patient's stay in the hospital. Evidence suggests that intensive, acute stroke rehabilitation is responsible for most of the recovery experienced by patients after a stroke. In the past, the process by which we assessed patients for rehabilitation was inconsistent. Patients were assessed and often placed in a subacute care setting where they had limited options for intensive acute stroke rehabilitation. Because of this traditional practice, the stroke unit and the acute rehabilitation unit developed a collaborative effort. This collaboration allowed for a multidisciplinary approach in developing a rehabilitation plan post-stroke, which evidence from studies has shown improves outcomes for stroke patients. Since the collaboration, the number of patients assessed for rehabilitation has increased, and the process has become more consistent. The number of stroke patients admitted to the acute rehabilitation unit has increased, which gives the patient the best shot at recovery.

The idea of collaborating with other team members caught on quickly. Not long after the development of the collaboration with the acute care unit and the stroke unit, multidisciplinary rounds were initiated on the stroke unit. By using a multidisciplinary approach to care of the patients in the hospital as well as to their discharge planning, the hospital can develop an individualized plan that includes patients, which increases the likelihood that they will adhere to the plan. Departments included in these rounds are nursing, social work, case management, physical therapy, speech therapy, occupational therapy, and clinical dieticians. During rounds, these included departments address all aspects of the patient's care, which assists the team in developing a comprehensive plan of care. Participation by all disciplines has increased, which eliminates the silo effect that often occurs in health care delivery. Patients who are recognized as high risk for having discharge complications are identified earlier, which assists the team in achieving the best patient and family outcomes by identifying and tackling barriers expeditiously. Communication and professionalism has improved among members of the health care team. Nurses have developed a sense of pride by playing an active role in their patient's plan of care, which has increased the quality of care that they deliver.

That remarkable group of stroke survivors that I mentioned early on has chosen to give something back to other stroke patients. Because a stroke can be a devastating, life-altering event, talking with someone who has shared the same feelings is sometimes helpful. A stroke peer mentorship program was developed after a discussion at one of the stroke support meetings. The survivors expressed a desire to "give the patient and their loved ones something we didn't have: someone to talk to." Several volunteers from the support group have undergone training and make regular visits to stroke patients while they are in the hospital. The program provides encouragement and hope to other stroke survivors and allows the mentor and stroke patient to share experiences, which benefits both the mentor and the patient. Evidence suggests that building relationships is beneficial while recovering from a stroke. The program establishes a resource early and provides support and promotes a positive outlook on recovery.

I think that nurses feel the greatest pride when we know that the care we provide impacts our community in a positive way, and perhaps we can think of several experiences where we truly felt great about what we did. We learn so much from our patients, and each interaction we have with them strengthens our practice. Having a relationship with the stroke community has been a gift to me both professionally and personally.

EBP Pearl

Involvement of multidisciplinary team members and patients in evidence-based care improves outcomes.

Falls Again? A Story Without End

–Sylvia M. Belizario, MEd, BSN, RN, CNRN
Georgetown University Hospital
Washington, DC

After reviewing the charts of all of the patients who fell in my unit during the summer of 1990, I observed some common patient characteristics, such as unsteady gait, visual deficits as a result of a stroke, confusion, lethargy, disorientation, and taking sedatives or psychotropic drugs. Many of them fell around toileting time. I created a preliminary profile based on the internal evidence that I gathered, which I shared with the staff during an inservice on falls that turned into several brainstorming sessions. The content of these sessions formed some of the groundwork for the development of our fall prevention program. By November 1990, under the direction of my supervisor, Ms. Norma Bent, and with two other nurse specialists, Ms. Margaret Brown and Ms. Marissa Rossoukh, we completed a fall prevention protocol with accompanying documentation forms, including a fall risk assessment, fall prevention checklist, patient care standard, patient care plan for the clinical information system, and fall alert list. In addition, we included fall alert stickers for the chart, patient's door, and head of the patient's bed.

I took the information back to the staff. After training them on the fall protocol and the use of the forms, the staff were eager to do the pilot in the unit because they knew that they were part of its development. By April 1991, based on the results of the pilot and the staff's feedback, we made revisions to the forms, such as including directions on the form itself on when to complete the fall risk assessment. We included, "To be completed on admission, transfer, at discharge, and every 3 days if the patient is high risk." We developed a focused review form to review every fall and a fall monitoring tool. All of these changes were reflected in the protocol. We implemented the fall prevention protocol with the revisions in my unit. In addition, we included other units in the fall prevention protocol, including the department of critical care, neuroscience, and emergency nursing. About a year later, we developed a Clinical Guideline for Fall Prevention that included more improvements in the protocol. Further, we added more items to the fall prevention flow sheet. As we continued to implement this protocol, the number of falls in the 36-bed neuroscience unit (9 neuro-ICU, 3 step-down, 24 general neuroscience) gradually decreased from a monthly fall rate of 5–6 to about 3–4 while the staff's adherence to the fall prevention protocol slowly improved. In August 1992, the Hospital Quality Assessment and Improvement Committee approved the fall prevention program with some recommendations. The staff was very proud and encouraged to see "neuroscience nurses" among the list of staff that developed the fall prevention protocol. They willingly piloted the revised protocol from September–October 1992.

The department of neurology formed a departmental quality assessment and improvement committee made up of the chairman of the neurology department; the neurology attending physicians, resident, and interns; a social worker; a representative from the Hospital Quality Assessment and Improvement Office and Utilization Review; a clinical manager; and me. I reported a summary of the focused review of falls from my unit monthly. In one of these meetings, I shared that a conflict was growing between the day and evening shift staff because the evening shift claimed that the day shift's fall risk assessment of some patients was always wrong. The day shift would assess the patient as a low fall risk, but when the evening shift arrived and completed their assessment, the patient would be reclassified as high risk for fall. The chairman of the department of neurology told me to go "figure it out." I had my suspicions about the reason that this was happening; however, I went back to reading the charts of these "problem patients," interviewing the staff, and reading some articles and textbooks. I realized that all the "problem patients" were stroke patients who experienced sundowning syndrome. Because of this, we completed our fall risk assessment not only on admission, transfer, every 3 days while the patient was at risk, and at discharge, but also "whenever the patient's condition changed." The charge nurses also included the number of high-risk patients in the 24-hour report that they completed every shift and submitted to the nursing supervisor (clinical service manager).

After piloting the protocol for 2 months, we changed the frequency of completing the fall prevention checklist to hourly instead of every 2 hours. The staff, both registered nurses and nursing assistants, had to work together to accomplish the hourly rounds. In addition, the Hospital Quality Assessment and Improvement Committee mandated that the fall prevention protocol be implemented throughout the entire hospital.

Three years after the implementation of the fall prevention protocol, a surge of falls occurred on my unit. From July through October 1993, 4–5 patients fell monthly with a total of 17 falls (about 13% of the number of admissions during that period). I reviewed the focused reviews on the falls and documentation. I watched the staff at different times of the day to observe what they did to implement the protocol and interviewed them. Were they doing their safety checks as they should? The major findings included lack of knowledge among the patients, family, and staff on falls and the fall protocol; lack of communication between staff and visitors; incomplete fall checklists; no consistent notification of the unit manager when falls occurred on the off shift; inconsistent marking of high-risk patients' names on the assignment sheet by charge nurses; and failure to consistently replenish the supplies of fall stickers and fall prevention checklists. I shared these observations at various staff meetings. I reminded staff about teaching patients and families regarding falls, specifically family members needing to let the nurses know when their visit was over and placing the side rails up before leaving. The secretaries made sure that fall stickers were on the charts of fall risk patients. The unit manager made the charge nurses accountable for completing the assignment sheets.

To increase and sustain the staff's awareness of the fall protocol, the unit manager and I made more frequent rounds to check on the staff's implementation of the protocol, especially the hourly rounds and placing fall alert stickers on doors and above the patients' beds. I checked the documentation of the hourly rounds on the fall prevention checklist. Lastly, I reviewed the final version of the fall prevention protocol with the staff and annually thereafter for the next few years while reinforcing their responsibility of implementing the protocol appropriately because it started in our unit. By May 1994, the number of falls decreased by 50% (8–9 falls) and by December 1994, the number of falls dropped by another 75% (0–2 falls).

When the nursing documentation committee completed updating and revising the nursing documentation forms in 1995, the initial fall risk assessment was incorporated into the patient database. The name of the fall prevention checklist was changed to "safety check flow sheet," and staff continued to document their hourly rounds on it. I presented this project as a poster at the Stroke Awareness Day at Howard University Hospital in March 1997. A few years later, Rachel Smith, PhD, of the Department of Nursing Professional Development and Performance Improvement initiated a hospital-wide fall committee made up of representatives from the medical staff, risk management, the Director of the Department of Nursing Professional Development and Performance Improvement, the pharmacy, the nurse manager, nursing staff, and me to review all the falls that happened in the hospital.

Between 2005 and 2008, during one of our mock surveys for the Joint Commission (JCAHO) preparation, Ms. Shirley Noah took a copy of our safety check flow sheet to show other hospitals that did not have one or that were just starting their own fall prevention programs.

The fall prevention program started small in 1990. It took approximately 2–3 years of continuously improving the protocol and its implementation processes before we had a finished product that was not only evidence-based, but highly successful. The observations and feedback of the bedside nurses, the doers of the protocol, and the end users of the tools were very valuable not only in getting this performance improvement project started but also in making improvements until its final version. Three nurse specialists worked on this project initially, but the direction and support provided by the supervisor was undeterred and encouraging, helping this project stay active and alive until it became a hospital-wide protocol.

Though many nursing actions were listed in the safety check flow sheet, I learned that not all actions would be applicable to every patient and that the most effective fall prevention strategy was the hourly rounds with teamwork. With the RNs and nursing assistants working together, the falls in my unit were maintained on a monthly average of 0–2 until a dramatic change in patient mix occurred that resulted in a decrease of neuroscience patients in the unit. The fall prevention protocol was still in place throughout the hospital until my departure in 2008.

EBP Pearl

Being observant and collecting internal data on the patients in your clinical practice setting can lead to practice changes that result in high-quality care and improved patient outcomes throughout an entire health care system.

Evidence-Based Practice in Primary Care

–Denise Boehm, MSN, RN, NE-BC
Associate Chief Nurse, Primary Care
VA Pittsburgh Healthcare System, Pittsburgh, Pennsylvania

The VA Pittsburgh Healthcare System (VAPHS) defines *professional development* as the continuous improvement in the quality of nursing care and practice. We support professional development by encouraging individual staff members to assess their learning needs, take action to improve their knowledge base, and continually evaluate their competence. VAPHS nurses are accountable and self-directed for their own personal and professional growth and development; this accountability extends to our patients, to each other, to VAPHS, and to the broader nursing profession. The continual search for improvement and implementation of best practices is made possible through our shared governance structure that supports nurses' autonomy, authority, and accountability for practice. The nurses of the primary care team have shown how they embrace shared governance and support veteran centered care (VCC) in the following example of shared governance at work.

Primary care is offered within all three of our unique VAPHS facilities. The Purple Team is the name of the primary care team at the Highland Drive facility. Highland Drive is a campus-style setting with many buildings, one of which is home to our inpatient acute psychiatry units, as well as mental health clinics, dental clinics, and the compensation and pension program. Because the setting is primarily that of acute inpatient and outpatient psychiatry, many of the resources within this campus are associated with the needs of that unique patient population. In 2008, the Highland Drive division no longer kept oxygen or any associated supplies on-site because a patient on oxygen did not meet admission criteria to inpatient psychiatry. Furthermore, medications and emergency supplies were limited to the emergency response teams. The nurses working in the Purple Team identified the potential problems that a patient with acute needs could have, such as the need for a nebulizer treatment. This identified patient care problem was brought to the Professional Practice Council (PPC). Using the shared governance model, the PPC chairperson, April Adame, BSN, RN, took the lead in seeing this to its resolution. She located established evidence-based standards of care for patients presenting to a primary xare clinic with oxygen needs. She then surveyed other VA primary care clinics as well as primary care clinics in the community to establish trends in practice. While doing these surveys, April also determined what level of providers within these clinical settings were administering nebulizer treatments if needed in a primary care setting. After completion of the surveys, she then conducted a literature review with the assistance of the VAPHS Chief of Library Services, Susan Hoehl.

April then compiled all of her data, developed an action plan, and presented first to the Purple Team PPC. With favor from the unit-based PPC, the recommendations were then forwarded to the facility-level Clinical Leadership Council (CLC). April outlined that her data supported having the resources to administer oxygen and nebulizer treatments in a primary care clinic should the need arise. Concurrence on this plan was achieved at CLC level and ultimately approved by the Nursing Administrative Leadership Council (NALC) as well. She then worked with the nursing educator, Virginia Manning, to train each nurse on the Purple Team on the proper technique to administer a nebulizer treatment. After competency of each nurse in primary care was documented, April worked with pharmacy and distribution to ensure that the supplies needed were available, thus successfully changing practice and establishing processes for safe, effective patient care.

Shared governance assists in developing a caring-healing practice that fosters partnerships, negotiation, coordination, and connection between nurses and others, especially veterans, other health care providers, and administration. Though shared governance is not necessarily a novel approach, it fosters those involved to work together to transform a dated system, offering new visions, creativity, and other possibilities not viewed as possible in the past. Shared governance is, in essence, a force for veteran-centered care. The primary care team, in keeping with our care delivery model of Veteran Centered Care (VCC), recognized that patients coming to the primary care clinic at the Highland Drive Division of VAPHS were at times in need of treatments not currently offered, worked through the processes, and as a result, delivered cutting-edge care second to none.

―――――――――◯―――――――――

EBP Pearl

External evidence from research plus internal evidence, combined with a clinician's expertise and patient preferences and values, leads to high quality evidence-based care.

The Heart of Hourly Rounding

–Kimberly Clark, MS, RN

–Felice Espinosa, MBA, BSN, RN

–Ma Jomela Nagal, MBA, BSN, RN

–Ruby De Jesus, BSN, RN, CPN

–Annis Felicien, BSN, RN

–Mary Gordon, PhD, RN, CNS-BC

Texas Children's Hospital, Houston, Texas

Hourly rounding is an evidence-based, practical approach toward providing quality customer service and engaging the patient/family in their daily care. Hourly nurse rounding gained momentum with the Studer Group when its research subsidiary, the Alliance for Health Care Research (AHCR), conducted a study of nursing units in several hospitals nationwide. The evidence showed that rounding on patients using keywords that focused on common patient needs (pain, positioning, potty and personal needs, and patient safety—referred to as the 4 Ps) demonstrated an increase in patient satisfaction scores by 12 mean points, decreased usage of patient call lights by 37.8%, and improved patient safety, such as falls by 50%.

Hourly rounding was piloted on the neurology/neurosurgery unit in July 2009 with the goals to decrease usage of patient call lights, improve overall patient satisfaction scores, promote patient safety, and provide the nursing staff with a model to cluster quality patient care. In 2009, patient/parent satisfaction scores on the neurology/neurosurgery unit were < 90% for the first three quarters, the number of calls on the call light during the first quarter was 2,950, and the unit had one of the highest patient fall rates in the hospital, 3.6 falls/1000 patient days.

Staff members were eager to embrace the new model and helped to develop education for implementation of new practices. Parent education flyers were developed and audit tools used to track compliance.

Both RNs and Patient Care Assistants (PCAs) played a vital part in hourly rounding. Training and educational materials were developed by the staff with the use of scripting (keywords at key times) to explain the process to the patient/family. During each patient admission, PCAs introduce themselves and their role to patient and family, update the whiteboard in each patient room with names of care providers for the shift and rounding time, and provide parents a copy of the Hourly Rounding Handout with a thorough explanation of the process.

The RN and PCA alternate hours to round, for example RN at odd hours and PCA at even hours. Rounding is performed every hour between 6:00 A.M. and 10:00 P.M. and every 2 hours between 10:00 P.M. and 6:00 A.M. Staff update the whiteboard with the current rounding time and initials. During this time, bedside routines are clustered and viewed as a bundle of interventions. Prior to leaving the room, staff asks, "Is there anything else I can do for you before I leave?"

As is true for any new process in our facility, assigned committee members perform random audits of whiteboards to verify they are updated. The leadership team interviews patients and families to validate staff's compliance and the effectiveness of the hourly rounding. Direct feedback is given to the staff at the time of audits. Each staff member is held accountable for their performance in a manner similar to performance initiative audits.

Not only did the unit achieve their goals with hourly rounding, but they achieved much more than expected with the parents. Parents verbalized their feelings of comfort knowing that somebody is there taking care of their children's needs. Today, they utilize hourly rounding as an opportunity to voice their concerns and raise clinical questions. Parents feel empowered because the nurses meet their needs promptly, and they view the nurses as their advocates. Hourly rounding has created a true health care partnership with the families. As one parent noted, they have good rapport with the nursing staff, which makes their stay in the hospital less stressful.

The hourly rounding process has had a positive impact on the nursing team and the nursing process. Patient care has become a collaborative team effort among the nurse, PCA, patient, and family. The parents are kept updated on the plan of care, and patients' needs are anticipated and met in a timely manner. Hourly rounding has also made the staff more aware of their patients' conditions, and they are alerted to triggers that may require further assessment and management.

One nurse shared that she became a believer in hourly rounding when she found the side rail down on the crib of her 7-month old patient and the parents had fallen asleep. She immediately raised the rail to prevent a fall or injury to the patient. She then used that moment to reinforce patient safety with the parents. She was so thankful that she entered the room to round and thought the consequences of not rounding could have been much worse. Another nurse shared that she became a believer in hourly rounding one night when she had a very busy patient assignment. Hours passed, and neither she nor anyone else had checked on her other patients. When she later went in to check on the patient, the IV had infiltrated. She felt that if she or her PCA had rounded on the patient, the magnitude of the infiltration could have been minimized.

Additional benefits of hourly rounding identified by the nursing staff include that it provides an organized approach to care delivery that ensures patients receive personal attention specific to their care needs, promotes positive relationships with patients and families, and facilitates a two-way communication that gives patients a sense of control about their care. One nurse felt that hourly rounding has had a considerable impact on holistic nursing and could revolutionize patients' insight about nurses playing a major role in optimizing their healing and autonomy.

The hourly rounding process provides nurses the assurance that patients are kept safe and comfortable by proactively meeting their needs, consequently decreasing the call light usage. The patients and families seem more willing to play an active role in their care as they realize that someone is available who can attend to their needs.

Because this process began on the unit a year ago, patient satisfaction scores have increased in 2010 to 90.1% for the fiscal year average. Patient falls have declined to 1.9 falls/1000 patient days. Patient call light usage decreased by 14% to 2,542 calls for the third quarter.

Hourly rounding brought an innovative, evidence-based approach to nursing care on the neurology/neurosurgery unit, bringing with it a renewed commitment to quality patient care because the staff knows they are making a difference in the lives of their patients. The patients and families recognize that they are an essential component of the health care team and seem willing to comply with care recommendations. The results of the hourly rounding process have led to changes in practice that have improved patient outcomes and patient-centered care.

EBP Pearl

Evidence-based interventions bring staff and family satisfaction and improved patient outcomes!

New Grads and Evidence-Based Practice: Let's Not Shock the Babies

–Amy Conway, RN
Diamond Children's Medical Center
Tucson, Arizona

In 2007, I was one of three new graduate nurses working in pediatric intensive care. We completed our summer externships together on the same unit and were thrilled with our new jobs. Though we felt well prepared for the challenges, we also were very humbled working alongside an amazing group of intelligent and experienced nurses.

During our first year, we participated in the University Health Care System/American Association of Colleges of Nursing (UHC/AACN) BSN Nurse Residency program. An evidence-based practice (EBP) project was required, and we were eager to do something relevant to our unit. At that time, some discussion on the unit between the pediatric intensivists and the nurses concerned peripheral nerve stimulation and "train-of-four."

Neuromuscular blockade (paralysis) is often used to facilitate mechanical ventilation when sedation with analgesia is not sufficient for eliminating respiratory effort. Prolonged weakness and paralysis are potential complications of this treatment. The goal of dosing and titrating the drip was to prevent spontaneous movement without completely blocking all muscular response. This approach would help to preserve muscle tone.

At that time, standard practice and our hospital protocol called for the use of peripheral nerve stimulation and train-of-four monitoring to determine the degree of neuromuscular blockade. The procedure involves placing electrodes over the area of the nerve (typically the ulnar nerve) and using a peripheral nerve stimulator to apply electrical current in a series of four consecutive stimuli (train-of-four). With no blockade, the muscle responds with a series of four twitches. The desired effect was two of four, indicating a partial blockade.

On our unit, the nurses had some concern that the effectiveness of the peripheral nerve stimulation was questionable. At times, even with troubleshooting equipment and verifying appropriate conditions, nurses observed no twitches in response to nerve stimulation, yet the baby would move spontaneously. If no response or twitches were seen with the initial 10 milliamps of current, the protocol called for increasing the current to 20, then to 40, and up to 80 milliamps. Though I generally believe "the protocol is our friend," this protocol seemed anything but friendly to our babies. Shocking the babies and ramping up the current when response was episodic at best posed an ethical dilemma. Our goal was to find evidence to support a change in practice that seemed more humane. If we observed movement while doing our other care procedures, could we avoid using the peripheral nerve stimulator?

The results of our investigation were scant. We contacted other hospitals to determine their protocols; those that responded were using a similar protocol and standard. In searching the literature, we found a wealth of articles on peripheral nerve stimulation describing why it is done, how to do it, and its potential complications, but we found nothing on alternatives.

Finally, we found a single paper that provided a glimmer of hope. It met most of the important criteria. It was peer-reviewed and authored by nurses. The study was conducted on critically ill pediatric patients, and the design was a controlled method comparison. The researchers looked at movement in response to other stimulation that was a necessary component of patient care (mouth care, eye care, and tactile stimulation of the abdomen/diaphragm area). The nurses found poor agreement between observed muscle movement and train-of-four scores during infusions of neuromuscular blocking agents, whereas better agreement was found after the infusions were discontinued. The study concluded that observation and assessment of the child's movements with other care procedures could be used in conjunction with peripheral nerve stimulation to determine an appropriate response to neuromuscular blocking agents.

The evidence from this single study allowed us to go forward and modify our hospital protocol. The suggested changes were well-received by our clinical practice committee that reviews and oversees all patient care protocols. Documentation of spontaneous or other movement could substitute for movement in response to nerve stimulation. While this might seem like a small change (and simply common sense), the experience was important for us in several ways.

In nursing school, our introduction to EBP was necessary, but academic. With tangible motivation from our unit and direct care experience, the process became more meaningful. With a clear question and goal, it was easy to sort through the papers and determine what was relevant to our situation. It was heartening and inspiring to discover research by other nurses that was driven by concerns similar to those of our staff members. Most importantly, it was empowering. Since this initial experience, I have yet to hesitate to suggest and follow through to make evidence-based changes when a protocol seems to have shortcomings.

EBP Pearl

Evidence-based practice empowers clinicians to make changes that improve patient outcomes.

Reveille! Time to Wake Up . . . Get Up: A Personal Journey With EBP

–Bertha L. Davis, PhD, RN, ANEF, FAAN
Professor of Nursing, School of Nursing
Hampton University, Hampton, Virginia

This story describes my personal journey through health care, a lived experience characterizing evidence-based practice. For decades, I had a problem with my foot shaking, caused by what I now know were Jacksonian seizures. One day, I left my office to go talk to the manager of our computer lab. Suddenly, while talking to her, I found myself leaning to my left side as if in slow motion, my speech fading as I was falling. I was amazed that the manager, a 120-pound, 5-foot tall female, was able to catch me in her arms. Just as she was laying me down, a colleague slid through the door as if gliding into home plate or landing a plane on a runway, her lap in position, to prevent my head from crashing to the floor. I was able to sit up after several minutes, but my right side was paralyzed. I went from the bright lights to darkness as I lay on the floor, unable to speak or move the right side of my body. I was transported by ambulance to the hospital. Although I did not lose consciousness and could see and hear, I could not speak.

After arriving in the emergency department (ED), I was able to move my right leg. I was seen by the ED nurse, who took a thorough history and asked if I previously had any neurological symptoms. The physician followed up and asked the same questions, and I confirmed the nurse's account of the history. The physician scheduled a computerized axial tomography (CAT) scan, and the nurse explained why it was needed. Another CAT scan with dye contrast was performed. I knew when the nurse explained a repeat CAT scan was needed that something suspicious was found on the initial scan. A nurse colleague I had known since college, and who had known my husband before we were married, talked with the physician who explained the situation to my husband. The colleague knew my husband would not take the news well. She focused his attention from the diagnosis to the fact that I had regained function on my right side, and I was able to talk normally. I knew the repeat scan would make my husband nervous, but my friend could handle him. I returned to the ED after the scan to a husband who was visibly shaken and repeatedly asking, "Are you all right?"

The nurse came in to provide the preliminary results and to say the physician would come and give specific findings. As the physician emerged from behind the curtain, I waited for the verdict. He indicated I had a tumor about the size of a quarter in the sagittal suture, which is located at the middle of the top of the head. The outcome was I needed surgery to remove the tumor, and it needed to be scheduled soon. The symptoms could return the next day, a week, or months from now, and surgery was imminent. Nurse colleagues and friends started finding experienced neurosurgeons. After deliberating, I decided on a neurosurgeon who had already studied my case and consulted with other neurosurgeons in the area.

I was given a furlough to get my affairs in order. The furlough included taking care of family and work responsibilities; having the general workup required for any major inpatient surgery—hospital, insurances, chemistries, and other scans to determine if changes had occurred since the ED visit; attending church; meeting family and close friends; undergoing a mental health consultation; and planning my discharge. The most important thing for me became prayer and my hospital attire post-op, and I interject this here because during the first days post-op, I could not don the clothing I had bought, but prayer was a constant companion.

The day came for surgery, and my husband transported me to the hospital. The nurses came in the holding area with a flurry of activity that made my husband even more anxious than he was initially. My friends were there, some to talk and pray with me and others to take care of my husband. Other friends made sure my son got to camp that day, who, at age 14, said before I left home, "I will see you after surgery." The nurses continued preparing me for surgery, and this included explaining advance directives and power of attorney documents that I signed immediately. My husband began fuming and asked why I had to sign the papers, not because he did not know about them, but because he was thinking about the possible outcome and that he might be required to use them. Friends went out of the room with him until he could get himself together. The use of evidence-based practice here suggests that meeting the specific needs of a family member may eliminate unnecessary anxiety.

I left for surgery and was in surgery for at least 4 hours, I was told, but what is instructive here is what was going on during the surgery—the inclusion of those who were waiting to hear news about my status. A nurse in the operating room (OR) was relaying the status of the surgery to the nurses in the waiting area, who were relaying the information to my friends, family, and colleagues. Finally, the surgery ended, and I was sent to recovery. I was asleep so long that the nurses became concerned because it was not easy to awaken me. Little did they know I was a deep sleeper and had not slept for 2 days before the surgery. My vitals were stable, so the hospital staff people—nurses and doctors—were not alarmed, but you know who was—my husband, so I am told. I was moved to the ICU and was startled by my friend who was sitting in a chair by the bed looking directly at me, waiting for me to wake up. She told the nurse I needed something for pain because I had not been given any medication since being in the ICU. My friend told me later that I said I did not need medication, but she told the nurse to give me something anyway. This is an example of how blending clinical expertise, research, and patient preferences can be used to provide the best evidence-based care.

After the first two days in the ICU, I opened my eyes more often, but could not speak or move independently. I was uncomfortable for several reasons: the compression splints on my legs were circulating air and made noise when filling up and going down; the tube from the drain site in my head was uncomfortable; the alarms in the ICU were constantly beeping; a patient was constantly calling out night and day for someone who was either not present or who she did not realize was present; the sun was shining for hours through the window in my face at varying intensities depending on the time of day; music was playing too loudly in my ear and included tunes I did not like; and nurses were talking to me but did not seem to understand that I wanted to speak, but could not. Further, when my speech was returning, the nurses would talk to me in an effort to meet my needs, I am sure, but they did not slow down long enough to hear my answers. Each time they would enter the room, it took the same amount of time for me to answer, so I was thinking to myself, "Oh no, there she goes again. Come back." I thank God I was not in pain. My experiences in the ICU demonstrate how often opportunities to apply evidence-based practice to decision-making are missed.

I managed to sit up on my own 2 days later, speak normally, and have the tube in my head removed. I was also moved out of the intensive care unit to a room on the floor. The function on my right side returned slowly, and I was sent to a local rehabilitation center. The rehabilitation center was not a place of rest; I had speech, recreational, occupational, and physical therapy 3 times a day. I was ordered not to get up without assistance and was observed when eating. One day, I thought I had progressed enough to get in the wheelchair and eat independently, so I decided to take things into my own hands. I successfully transported myself from the bed to the wheelchair, but when I got myself to the sink in the bathroom and attempted to stand on my right side, I slipped back into the chair. After I finished brushing my teeth, I began eating and almost choked. I then realized that the orders were given for a reason, and I now had my own evidence to support the importance of obeying the instructions of the health care team. I spent several weeks in rehab getting much-needed therapy, including learning how to get from the floor to a chair, walk with a cane up and down stairs, and drive a car with my left foot. Thanks to the evidence-based care I received from the many providers who helped me to develop all of these skills that I still use today, 14 years later, my motto is, "Reveille: Time to Wake Up . . . Get Up!"

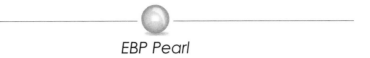

EBP Pearl

You never know the impact your role in providing evidence-based care can make in the lives of patients.

EBP: Not Just a Buzzword

–Linda D. Denton, MSN, RNC
University of North Carolina Health Care
Children's Hospital Newborn Critical Care Center, Chapel Hill, North Carolina

Evidence-based practice is a buzzword in the nursing community. Any nurse who has ever revised policies or worked on a unit practice committee is familiar with the phrase, but do we actually look at the evidence to guide our practice? Or are we led by customs and individuals' anecdotal experience? The answer to that question for our Level III neonatal intensive care unit is a resounding, "Yes, we look at the evidence!" A wonderful example of this is a quality improvement project that is presently going on in our unit.

In the interest of transparency, I need to say that my coworker J.B. and I entered into this project with absolutely no idea about what we were getting into. Yes, we had volunteered for a Six Sigma Green Belt project, and we knew that it would be some kind of quality improvement effort. But the places that this would take us, the depth and breadth of the project, and the amazing outcomes of the endeavor were things we could not even begin to imagine.

At the start, we didn't know what would be addressed in our quality improvement project. Our medical director, and project sponsor, had chosen two initiatives: (1) improving the discharge process, and (2) decreasing catheter-associated blood stream infections (CABSIs). By fate or luck of the draw, J.B. and I ended up on the CABSI project. I didn't even know what the letters stood for at the time. Our third teammate was J.K., a neonatal nurse practitioner who had already been doing a lot of CABSI work. She was head of the unit practice committee, which was deemed the C.S.I. (Combating Systemic

Infections) committee and had been tracking and working on decreasing central line infections.

As the three of us went through the Six Sigma Green Belt classes, we had to identify our goals and what we were going to measure, brainstorm possible causes of CABSIs, and propose interventions and solutions—then the real work began. We learned that we couldn't just assume or guess what the causes might be and what could correct them. We actually had to collect internal evidence (i.e., practice data) to demonstrate what was going on with central lines. We conducted discreet observations of staff members while maintaining and accessing central lines. From these observations, we counted the number of times per day that each of our central lines was accessed. We requested that nurses complete surveys to gather further information. We timed nurses while they were trying to locate our hospital's central venous access device (CVAD) policy on the hospital intranet and asked them their opinions on the policy. We did a focus group with physicians and neonatal nurse practitioners. We conducted literature searches in online databases and read and reread the studies we could find about CABSIs. General (adult-based) central line "bundles" and other recommendations to improve care were readily available in the literature. This was all good, but we wanted specific neonatal research. Because of the paucity of published neonatal studies, we also benchmarked against similar units in the state who had made practice changes and achieved positive outcomes.

After reviewing most of the evidence, we noted that the standard CABSI outcome measurement was *infections per catheter days*. However, given that the major participants in central line maintenance are nurses, we chose to use something more concrete and more meaningful to them as our prime outcome measurement, which was *days between infections*. Our nurse practitioner teammate put a project whiteboard on the unit and started a running count of days between infections. She updated the board frequently with the information she received from the infection control department. Nurses were encouraged to check the board frequently for progress.

To facilitate a successful outcome, we decided to focus our actions on two different concepts: (1) education, and (2) buy-in. The education facet is self-explanatory. The buy-in solutions were aimed at helping nurses realize the vital importance of using proper aseptic technique each time they accessed a central line. Further, we emphasized the impact that any single CABSI has on the infant, the family, the staff, the medical providers, and the hospital. To further focus nurses' attention on the project, we developed unit-specific guidelines for central line maintenance, 2 videos, and about 15 illustrated "slogan" reminder signs for posting around the unit.

We made several important practice changes based on the CABSI "bundles" recommendations and our benchmarking. We sent e-mails, talked to nurses face-to-face, presented updates at staff meetings, and asked for and received feedback from the staff. One of the most powerful interventions we used was a video made by the father of a baby who had died as a result of a CABSI. His goal in sharing his story was for nurses and medical providers to be so moved that they would change their practice in ways that would decrease the chance that another family would have to go through what his had, which, gauging staff responses, seemed to be met.

During the many years that central line infections in the unit had been tracked, the longest recorded period between CABSIs was about 70 days. For the most part, a typical bedside nurse didn't really pay much attention to the incidence of central line infections unless it happened to be her/his baby who had a septic work-up and initiation of antibiotics. The general attitude of the unit was that of *inevitability*—critically ill premature babies who had central lines for weeks to months were at high risk for CABSI and nothing could be done to prevent it. The evidence directly countered this assumption, and we demonstrated that since we conducted evidence-based interventions, the assumption had not been supported on our unit as well. After the initial rollout of the practice changes, our unit had 199 infection-free days! This far surpassed our goals, and even some of our dreams. Though certainly everyone was disappointed and saddened that an infant had become septic, celebrations were held on the unit to recognize the accomplishment of a record number of infection-free days. Furthermore, we wanted to thank the staff for their cooperation. Of course, we started over at "0" infection-free days after that baby's infection was confirmed; however, we reached about 116 days before another infant was diagnosed with a CABSI.

It has been well over a year since we began our Six Sigma classes, which prompted gathering internal and external evidence. Given that none of us initially knew what we were getting into when we volunteered for the Green Belt project, I can honestly say that it has been the most interesting and the most rewarding endeavor of my 27-year nursing career. To consider that even *one* baby's life might have been saved by our efforts is more than enough to make the year of work worthwhile.

Another aspect of the project that was both surprising and gratifying was the attitude of the staff and the change in our *inevitable* unit culture. During this past year, the nursing staff have been amazing. We have had none of the usual grumblings about changes in practice. Instead, people look at the evidence presented and accept what needs to be done. Seeing that teamwork and professionalism and being a part of an initiative that has brought such awesome outcomes makes it easy to go on from here. The project itself may come to an end, but this unit will never be the same. We will continue practice based on evidence so that our babies and families have quality care, and we will work toward our goal of zero infections! Acknowledgements: Special thanks to the nursing staff and medical providers of UNC NCCC and to my teammates: JoeBeth Bongares-Brown, BSN, RN, and Joanne Kilb, MSN, RN, NNP.

EBP Pearl

Evidence-based change is sustainable, impactful change. JUST DO IT!

Evidence-Based Practice Leads to Cultural Awareness

–Dawn R. Horak, MSN, RN
John C. Lincoln Hospital North Mountain
Phoenix, Arizona

Evidence-based practice is an approach to care that has influenced the way I practice, not only at the bedside but as a thought process to utilize in mentoring others who want to make a difference for their patients. I am a registered nurse who has been practicing for 25 years in a variety of areas of nursing including the emergency department (ED), risk/quality management, and in clinical education, all areas where outcomes might have a different focus, but all are patient- and family-centered. In my various roles, I have utilized evidence-based practice to support processes, change protocols, and improve safety/outcomes for patients and their families. After participating in an evidence-based practice fellowship, I found that my viewpoint that had once been task-driven had changed to a new focus—how I take care of patients today.

In the clinical educator role, I was asked to create a list of common phrases that could assist clinical staff with communicating with Spanish-speaking patients. This simple task turned into an indirect journey of learning about evidenced-based practice. As I began selecting key phrases, I found that every clinical area had their own perspective for what phrases should be on a standardized list. The list became too long to fit into your pocket, so I needed evidence to support which phrases were really necessary to improve the caregiver/patient experience.

As I began my journey, I sought to find others who had faced similar challenges. Our group, diverse in role, nationality, and perspective, brought many opinions up for discussion. Our common ground was that each one of us had worked clinically at the bedside and interacted with Spanish-speaking patients in the ED. We felt a need to increase cultural competence in the ED and across all levels of care at the hospital. As we began to look for research evidence, we began to see that our topic was broad and that we would need to "narrow it down," much like is achieved through writing a PICOT question. We continued to search for keywords that would lead us in the right direction, but found that culturally competent care had many components that included self-awareness, attitudes about culture, communication style, knowledge about culture, and cultural sensitivity. *Narrow it down* became the three little words that we heard several times over the next few months as we began to search for evidence about our topic. We discovered that Spanish is spoken by many cultures, and the Southwest comprises several cultures who speak Spanish with several dialects. In our search, we found that we needed assistance from our medical translators to help "narrow it down" to a specific culture. Based on demographic admissions data and translator interactions with patients, we chose the Hispanic population.

As our group worked toward consensus about the direction and outcome we wanted, we found that staff input was essential in determining the difference that would be made by communicating in the native language of Spanish-speaking patients. Staff responses to our questions about what would bring meaning centered on phrases that enhanced communication (i.e., greetings, performing interventions, and complaint follow-up).

They also identified that having more knowledge about health care beliefs and practices would enhance the patient/caregiver experience. The ED, respiratory therapy, and surgery were the areas in need of language augmentation; the focal area became the ED. We were all familiar with this area and felt that this was a point of entry for many Hispanic patients in seeking care and a great place to introduce the list of phrases.

Even though resources limited the scope of the project, we began to discuss the purpose of our project with others, and we found the cultural competence within our organization wonderfully cultivated the fertile ground for the project. Our efforts for initial staff education increased cultural awareness with the assistance of the medical translation interpreters. Our educational program provided an opportunity for staff to learn about beliefs and practices of the Hispanic population, which helped the staff to effectively problem solve when faced with this population of patients.

After leaving the ED, I returned to the bedside, where I have found that I now have a better understanding for what really is important to patients and their families who are Hispanic. I often reflect on my experiences and ponder how evidence-based practice can lead your thinking in many different directions, indeed; many that you might never have considered.

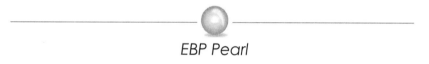

EBP Pearl

Evidence-based practice is about the effort extended to find the best evidence and combine it with clinician expertise and patient preferences. The joy is in the journey and its associated outcomes, not in the destination of saying, "We've done EBP"!

An Evidence-Based Practice Initiative in Progress

–H. Lynne Kennedy, MSN, RNFA, CNOR, CLNC
Inova Fair Oaks Hospita
Fairfax, Virginia

Evidence-based practice (EBP) is the conscientious integration of the best research evidence with clinical expertise and patient preferences in practice decision-making. As an operating room nurse, I noticed that gynecologists, who were the original developing group of laparoscopic surgery in the 1970s, still perform most of their surgical procedures nationwide using open techniques. This left patients in the hospital for several days, depleted of energy, and in pain for 6 to 8 weeks following routine surgery. Minimally invasive techniques may require a hospital stay of only a few hours with a substantially reduced recovery of 1 to 2 weeks. Since I was approaching the age where I also could be effected by surgical approaches in hysterectomy, and having watched so many patients over my nursing career experience pain when there existed other choices and other outcomes than an open operative procedure, I set up an appointment with the Chair of the Department of Gynecology at Inova Fair Oaks Hospital.

The problem was that patients were not receiving this evidence-based care because most practicing gynecologists around the United States do not possess the necessary skills to perform major surgery endoscopically. Though other surgical specialties adopted the minimally invasive approach as the standard, currently practicing gynecologists had been trained to use open techniques, particularly facilitating caesarian sections.

An educational program was developed that fit the professional and personal lifestyles of practicing physicians to help them to learn and excel with modern techniques and new skills. The series of courses and a mentorship program that provided a platform for practicing physicians was developed by the first assistant, a registered nurse with a background in education, and the chair of the department of gynecology, who had a burning desire to learn the techniques himself. The main objectives of the program were to improve the surgical experience for patients, to improve patient satisfaction, to improve physician satisfaction, to facilitate early discharge from the hospital with a quick recovery from surgery, and to reduce surgical costs.

The program was very successful in reducing the rate of minimally invasive surgeries conducted, with gynecologists performing 25–32% minimally invasive cases prior to the program (close to the national average in the United States), and 92% of gynecology cases performed using minimally invasive techniques after the program. Evidence-based practice can be successful with an interdisciplinary team! Now minimally invasive hysterectomy is the norm at Inova Fair Oaks Hospital.

With this evidence-based change come more questions. Thermal therapy has been used effectively in postpartum patients for many years; however, these products have not been used for gynecology surgical patients and specifically not for minimally invasive gynecological surgical patients. Regardless of the minimally invasive techniques used during this type of surgery, post-anesthesia care unit (PACU) nurses are responsible for managing the frequent perineal and abdominal pain patients experience postoperatively. Each PACU patient is assessed for pain level and treated accordingly with medications ordered by the physicians prior to surgery. Patients requiring parenteral narcotics cannot ambulate postoperatively for a minimum of a half hour. Patients requiring nonnarcotic pain medications can ambulate when their vital signs are stable. Criteria for discharge from PACU to second stage PACU for release home adds that the patient must desire to ambulate.

Patients experience a cascade effect of pain leading to delayed ambulation, leading to taking pain medications, leading to dizziness and nausea resulting in more pain from bladder spasms, and so it goes in perpetual motion unless nurses intervene. Knowing that pain medications were a part of the process that could stop the cascade, I began looking for methods of reducing pain in minimally invasive gynecology with a noninvasive nursing intervention. To find the answer to my question, I conducted a search for the evidence, but could not find a possible solution to the problem documented in peer-reviewed literature.

Currently, marketed products for postpartum cold thermal use exist, including cold packs (cold peri-pads [CPPs]) that are designed to alleviate the pain from soft tissue damage. The CPP application is done easily, can be adjusted by the patient for maximum comfort, and is inexpensive to use. These pads are safer than using ice packs, which are prohibited in many institutions, including the Inova Health System, because of the increased risk of skin damage. Evidence shows that using ice for 15–20 minutes can cause further damage to the tissues than already exists, including frostbite. Furthermore, studies have demonstrated in sports medicine that use of direct contact with ice can lead to severe frostbite. The CPPs were designed to prevent this type of unintended outcome, but reduce swelling while sustaining temperature. These pads are constructed as a pouch within a pouch. By squeezing as directed and rupturing the inner pouch, liquid and chemicals mix causing an immediate temperature change. Peri-Cold, a cold peri-pad (product of Hospital Marketing Services, Naugatuck, Connecticut) gradually and comfortably provides therapeutic cold to the perineum. The combination of cold and padding prevents direct skin contact, thereby preventing frostbite to the adjacent tissues, and it also sustains temperature for up to 40 minutes.

Given that I could find no definitive evidence to address how effective cold packs would be with postpartum women, I proposed a research study to evaluate a PACU nursing intervention using CPP applied to the perineum as soon as the patient enters the PACU. Outcomes would be postoperative pain and postoperative use of narcotic medication. Following approval of our Institutional Review Board (IRB), the study began. I expected to find that Laparoscopic Assisted Vaginal Hysterectomy (LAVH) surgical patients who received the CPP application would have lowered pain perception and not require narcotics, shorter time to ambulation, and shorter post-operative length of hospitalization than patients who did not receive the CPP intervention.

Though the study is still in progress, the results of this study are helping to build the body of knowledge of how to decrease pain scored in LAVH patients postoperatively. We are continuing to evaluate whether decreased pain for LAVH patients postoperatively results in decreased narcotic use, improved patient satisfaction, improved time to ambulation, improved time to urinate, and/or decreased length of hospital stay. Preliminary results show significant differences in that CPP applications impact the use of narcotics for the LAVH surgical patients.

EBP Pearl

Clinical expertise assists with application and generation of external evidence (i.e., research)!

Family Support During Resuscitation of a Loved One

–Deb Kramlich, MSN, RN, CCRN
Assistant Professor of Nursing, Saint Joseph's College of Maine
Cardiac Surgery Database Coordinator, Maine Medical Center, Raymond, Maine

Imagine being an experienced critical care nurse, the nurse in the family who everyone looks to for advice, comfort, and reassurance. Imagine one of your loved ones being acutely ill, facing frightening and life-altering decisions. You're getting vague information from the staff, and your gut tells you something isn't right. You follow your instincts, call the rest of the family, and arrive at the hospital, only to find your loved one has just been resuscitated. You're ushered to the bedside to find your loved one is conscious but intubated and is shaking her head "*no,*" indicating she wants no further intervention. And then, before any discussion can occur, before any decisions can be made, the unthinkable happens—another cardiac arrest. Where would you want to be?

That was my situation nearly 20 years ago when my grandmother, my rock and my role model, suffered her final cardiac arrest. I was physically removed from her bedside as she deteriorated; the door was closed in my face, not to be reopened until the resuscitation team emerged to tell us she had passed on. I knew she didn't want the resuscitation, and she didn't want to be alone. I felt utterly helpless, a foreign experience for someone who prided herself on being a leader. I felt I'd failed the person who had always supported me. I promised that one day I would find the means to make sure other patients and families wouldn't suffer a similar experience.

Over the years I found ways to allow families to remain with their loved ones during the most vulnerable times, often bending established norms and risking my colleagues' discomfort and disagreement. Still, I felt dissatisfied with the unpredictable approach to "family-centered care." I searched for opportunities to create an environment of consistent, unconditional acceptance of family presence.

Several years ago, following two particularly emotional resuscitations, I felt an urgency to step up those efforts. The first situation involved a young child whose parents were allowed to remain at the bedside, but for whom no support staff was available until after the child had died. It was difficult to comfort the family while I was actively involved in trying to save their child's life. In the second incident, a very large family completely disrupted the entire ICU because staff was unprepared and overwhelmed. Staff had agreed to allow a limited number of family members into the resuscitation, but had not anticipated the family's extreme reaction. It was clear that the practice of family presence during resuscitation was becoming more widely accepted, but staff expressed dissatisfaction with the lack of a formal structure and guidelines for supporting the families.

I was in graduate school at the time and had just completed both a research course and the evidence-based practice program offered by my institution. My employer also offered an annual sabbatical for nurses to complete an evidence-based practice project. Family presence was appearing more frequently in the scientific evidence. Our institution had adopted a patient- and family-centered care philosophy. The potential dedicated time to focus on a project seemed to be the perfect opportunity for my dream to become a reality. I applied for and was awarded the sabbatical to develop guidelines for family presence during resuscitation.

I assumed the institutional climate was ready for this type of practice change, and it would be a matter of just searching for and applying the evidence. Unfortunately, I was quite naive and sadly mistaken! I had done a thorough search and critical appraisal of the literature, and I decided to use the program developed by the Emergency Nurses Association as a template for my project. I distributed the multidisciplinary staff assessment tool to evaluate knowledge and attitudes regarding family presence. I had not predicted the intensity of emotional responses from many of the respondents. I realized I would need a strong team of mentors and advisors to accomplish my goals. This team would include opinion leaders from nursing, medicine, social work, pastoral care, clinical ethics, and various other ancillary departments. I also decided to invite several of the strongest opponents to participate, which turned out to be a very wise choice!

I knew it would be important to include the voice of the family in the development of the guideline, so I interviewed a number of family members to better understand their experience. I was fortunate to receive a small research grant from our local chapter of Sigma Theta Tau International to cover expenses such as travel, equipment, and transcription services. I spoke with spouses, adult children, and parents. I included families with a variety of experiences: those who had been present and those who had chosen not to be present; families whose loved one had survived and others who weren't so fortunate; and families whose experience was as good as it could possibly be as well as the opposite. It was emotionally draining, yet gratifying, as these families shared some of the most intimate details with me, reliving times of anguish and deep sorrow. Yet they were all thankful to be able to share their stories in the hopes of improving outcomes for other families. One exceptionally articulate family member even agreed to participate on the multidisciplinary guideline development team to make sure we "got it right."

Word quickly spread that the guideline development process was underway, and we found ourselves with requests from "guests" to attend meetings to express their concerns. Realizing the futility of closing the meetings, we built in time for anyone wishing to comment. Their remarks reflected the fears published in the literature: disruptive or psychologically traumatized families, negative effects on team performance, and increased litigation. They also feared loss of control, that a policy would be created requiring family presence at all resuscitations. As their anxieties were relieved, attendance at the "comment and concern" portion of the meetings soon dropped off, and we could focus on guideline development.

We used a very methodical and painstaking approach to developing the guideline. It was often tedious; sometimes all we accomplished during a meeting was the change of a word or phrase to satisfy everyone. Occasionally things got a little contentious, but we always had mutual respect as we kept our objectives in mind. It was important to the success of the project that we achieve consensus on every detail.

My sabbatical year was quickly coming to a close, and we finally had a workable guideline to pilot in our critical care units. I held my breath as implementation day approached, wondering if all my work would be for naught. We had a few glitches to work out in those early days, things like pagers not working and staff uncertain of the process. Soon, though, the calls, e-mail messages, and hallway conversations started coming: "I just have to tell you about the code on our unit and how much the family appreciated being there."; "We had our first family-witnessed code, and I was nervous, but it went smoothly."; "When can we start having family presence at our codes?" The positive responses were beyond my wildest dreams! It was so encouraging, in fact, that just 6 months after the pilot project was initiated, the guideline was approved for full implementation by institutional leadership at all levels.

It has been 2 years since the guideline was adopted, and it has become part of our organizational culture. Some of my most zealous opponents have embraced the evidence-based change. Departments from other campuses have requested education, and I recently trained a large group of nursing assistants to serve as family support staff. I continue to get unsolicited feedback from staff regarding their positive experiences and the gratitude from families.

This practice change has gone beyond the boundaries of our institution as I've presented my experience at local, regional, and national conferences. The guideline has been published on the Virginia Henderson International Nursing Library website as a Magnet best practice. Other hospitals in our parent health system have requested assistance with implementation of similar programs. I've also shared my experience and the guideline when requested on several practice Listserves as well as through telephone consultations. The most recent request came from one of the Canadian provinces as they develop family-centered practices on a provincial level. I pondered the impact of an observation; my dream had attracted international attention!

What began as a personal mission nearly two decades ago has resulted in a sustained evidence-based change with positive outcomes for patients, families, and practitioners. I can't help but think my grandmother's hand has been guiding me along this journey. Though I couldn't be with her during her transition, I have been able to give that gift to many other families. This would not have been possible without the many mentors who taught me how to engage in evidence-based practice and other brave predecessors who paved the way. I feel I've accomplished my life's work, and I am grateful beyond words.

EBP Pearl

Be persistent, dream, and engage—your patients, their families, and your colleagues will thank you for it!

Best Practice for Pain Identification in Cognitively Impaired Nursing Home Residents

–Christina Sacoco Manibog, MS, RN, RAC-CT
Leahi Hospital, Hawaii Health Systems Corporation, Honolulu, Hawaii
With support from the Hawaii State Center for Nursing

Often elderly patients suffer in silence. They don't want to burden family, friends, or caregivers, or they might be unable to express discomfort. This can become a major issue for seniors living at home or in the community, as well as for residents in nursing homes, especially those that are cognitively impaired. Nurses are concerned about underrecognizing signs and symptoms of pain in their elderly patients and are vitally interested in identifying a best practice for assessment.

A team of nurses from a Honolulu-based long-term care facility chose this problem for their evidence-based practice (EBP) project in March of 2009. The team had just completed a 2-day workshop sponsored by the Hawaii State Center for Nursing, led by nationally recognized creator of the Iowa Model for EBP, Marita Titler, PhD, RN, and Director of Research at The University of Hawaii School of Nursing and Dental Hygiene (UHSONDH), Debra Mark, PhD, RN. By investigating how other practitioners in similar situations assess their patients, the team sought to learn what might be appropriate in their facility, and they also realized that it could assist them in developing a clear problem statement for their project. The first step, then, was to conduct an evidence search, a process that had been taught in the workshop. An evidence review confirmed:

- Challenges to successfully evaluating and managing pain may include communication difficulties due to illness or language and cultural barriers, stoicism about pain, and cognitive impairment.

- It is a challenge to assess and manage pain in individuals who have cognitive impairment or communications difficulties.

- Nurses are the key to effective pain management; however, studies have demonstrated that nurses lack the pain knowledge necessary to manage their residents' pain effectively.

- The need exists for the establishment of a formalized system-wide interdisciplinary approach to pain management.

Though challenged by what they had learned, the team was undaunted in their desire to develop a best practice for pain assessment in the elderly cognitively impaired population. The team established a standardized, multidisciplinary approach to pain management to optimize resident outcomes. Key decision points that the team considered in selecting the Pain Assessment in Advanced Dementia (PAINAD) Scale were criteria and associated indicators used in the evaluation of tools for assessing pain in nonverbal elders as established by the City of Hope Pain & Palliative Care Resource Center. To ensure successful implementation of the practice change, a Pain Assessment educational program was designed to accommodate for culture/language differences to (a) promote better understanding about pain management and the use of pain assessment tools; (b) correct common misconceptions and myths about pain; and (c) provide education for staff that can allow them to recognize and be more sensitive to their resident's signs and symptoms of pain. The didactic content was delivered via interactive lectures and demonstrations; case studies were used as the basis for group discussions, practical exercises, and small group work.

The PAINAD tool, comprehensive pain assessment form, and pain monitoring flow sheet, were piloted house-wide for 60 days with all licensed nursing staff who care for cognitively impaired residents. As a result of the pilot, necessary modifications were made to the EBP guideline, and the change in practice was instituted by:

- Revising the pain policy and procedure

- Implementing the modification house-wide by providing additional inservices as appropriate to all clinical staff

- Continuing to perform quarterly chart audits and on-the-spot review/evaluation with staff as necessary

- Providing visual reminders and other resources for staff

To integrate the practice change permanently into nursing practice, the guideline and pain program/curriculum will be incorporated in the nursing orientation and then offered annually to the nursing staff thereafter, or as necessary.

Evaluation of the program included:

- Chart audits to determine nursing staff's documentation compliance

- Informal qualitative feedback regarding factors that facilitated and/or hindered the implementation of the pain assessment guideline

- Validation of the nursing staff's pain assessment through skilled competency

- Modification of the guideline based on the results

The results of the quality improvement initiative demonstrated an improvement in the quality and consistency in pain assessment and documentation:

- 71% improvement in completion of the Comprehensive Pain Assessment Form (for residents with cognitive impairment)

- 9% improvement in documentation of nonverbal indicators—upon implementation of PAINAD scale and pain monitoring flow sheet

- 40% improvement in documentation of pain location

- 11% improvement in documentation of pain intensity

- 55% improvement in documentation of assessment of interventions that improve pain

- 51% improvement in the consistent use of pain scale/observation method—upon implementation of PAINAD scale

- 9% improvement in care plan completion

- 33% improvement in inclusion of nondrug interventions in care plan

- 60% improvement in monitoring for analgesic side effects—upon implementation of pain monitoring flow sheet

In conclusion, to sustain the practice, the team recommended to (1) continue to educate staff and reinforce use of the new/revised assessment forms (PAINAD, Comprehensive Pain Assessment, and pain monitoring flow sheet) and (2) conduct monthly audits on appropriate use of PAINAD assessment form (for residents with cognitive impairment/communication difficulties) and pain monitoring flow sheet (for all residents) with signs and symptoms of pain and names of residents who are on routine/PRN meds.

EBP Pearl

Plan well and execute the EBP process!

Enhancing Inspiration: Nurses' Experiences With Project Enhance

–Alexis Matthews, BSN
MSG Student, University of Southern California, Camarillo, California
Intern, Coordinating Center of the Centers for Disease Control and Prevention-Healthy Aging Research Network (CDC-HAN), University of Washington and Senior Services, Seattle, Washington

It works. That is the consensus of responses from nurses when asked about the evidence-based program Project Enhance. To gain an understanding of nurses' experiences with Project Enhance, phone interviews with seven nurse volunteers who are currently involved in Project Enhance were conducted. This program is disseminated by Senior Services in Seattle, Washington, and targets older adults. It is divided into two interventions: EnhanceFitness and EnhanceWellness. The former is a physical fitness program that involves warm-up, cardio, strength training, cool-down, and stretching to keep older adults physically fit, strong, flexible, and active. EnhanceWellness is a program designed to help older adults reach their goals for improving their health and quality of life. Participants set an end goal that they want to reach within 6 months, and the EnhanceWellness team aides them in constructing an action plan to achieve that goal. In the mid-1990s, studies on the nascent forms of the EnhanceFitness and EnhanceWellness programs were conducted and demonstrated the numerous evidential benefits of each. Since then, both of these programs have been disseminated across the country, with new sites being established each year. Within these programs, nurses are employed in numerous levels of administration, from direct relations with participants to program supervision.

Some nurses, such as Suzanne Leveille, were involved in the original studies that produced the current programs established today. As one of the developers of the program, Leveille experienced Project Enhance in its earliest forms. She describes the reason why the idea for Project Enhance came to fruition: "We were very much interested in the notion of empowering patients for self-management." Therefore, Leveille and the rest of the collaborative team came together to choose components that would be most beneficial in enabling the elderly to maintain a healthy, active lifestyle. For example, it was decided that a nurse and a social worker were the proper choices for the roles of key interventionists. While Leveille was conducting the study, she and her team were able to adjust and modify the program to ensure the best possible outcomes for participants. Nurses who work with Project Enhance indicate that one of the major benefits of an evidence-based program is that many of the deficiencies have already been worked out by the time it is implemented. When programs are evidence-based and, therefore, have somewhat predicable outcomes, nurses are confident that these programs, such as Project Enhance, will yield successful outcomes for their participants.

One aspect of the Project Enhance program that did not turn out as expected was physician involvement. Originally the team thought that they would work closely with primary care physicians to work on participants' action plans. However, the team soon realized that though physicians were incredibly supportive of the programs, they did not consider it part of primary care because it was outside of the primary care environment. Nevertheless, this realization aided the true purpose of EnhanceWellness because it allowed the focus to be on empowering patients to involve their doctors with any concerns, questions, or updates.

Other nurses within the program confirmed that patients are often hesitant to speak up with their doctors, merely remaining passive in their treatment. EnhanceWellness promotes the belief that people must be active participants in their care. Another alteration made to the program in the beginning was the extent to which interventionists needed to promote physical activity. Leveille explained, "We also realized fairly early on that it was going to take a pretty aggressive amount of encouragement to get people onboard with the exercise components." This notion was incorporated into the program and resulted in improvements in participant cooperation in regards to exercise.

After Project Enhance was ready for dissemination, nurses all over the country began working for the program. Throughout their experiences, nurses have seen the overwhelming benefits for participants firsthand. Many of them described stories to me that were particularly inspirational. Elaine McMahon of the Partnership for Healthy Aging described one man who she remembered as having benefited immensely from this program. This man suffered from multiple lifelong chronic conditions, including congenital problems, being prone to falls, and a seizure disorder. He also was a heavy smoker. He was incredibly isolated; the only person he had contact with was his 90-year-old mother who lived close by. Because of his many health problems, he had been in and out of the hospital his whole life. After he learned of the success other people had experienced through EnhanceWellness, he began to believe that he could find some success as well. After completing the program twice, he had not been admitted into the hospital, he no longer smoked (a habit he was sure he would never break, prior to participating), and his self-health rating improved from fair to very good. Moreover, he found senior housing for both his mother and himself that was close to public transportation and allowed him to have more social interaction. He was also exercising almost every day. All of these improvements also led him to reduce his score on the Geriatric Depression Scale from 8 to 2 out of 15. McMahon still recalls how amazed and proud she was of this man's progress, even though it was years ago that he participated in EnhanceWellness. McMahon has witnessed many such stories and proclaims that "watching and being a part of supporting people who are going through this kind of change and improving their health and well-being was such an honor."

Sharon Congleton, a managing nurse at the Philadelphia Corporation for Aging, remembered a couple of participants of EnhanceFitness who saw tremendous results from the program. One woman began the program using a walker. She was also overweight and at high risk for falling. Through the program, the woman grew stronger, most importantly in her lower extremities, and gained a steadier gait. Because of her progress, the woman lost weight and moved around without the use of a walker or a cane. Another woman who Congleton recalled as having demonstrated significant improvement was one who had recently suffered a stroke prior to starting EnhanceFitness. Because of her stroke, she had left-sided weakness and needed to use a cane on her right side to get around. This woman did not believe that anything could be done about her issues and thus neglected her left side, contributing to her weakened state. At first, she could only do the in-chair version of the exercise regimen. As she became stronger, she did the exercises while holding onto the chair. Eventually she completed each class standing completely on her own. She had gained back strength on her left side and a new sense of confidence.

These stories are only some of the countless others that nurses expounded upon with pride and awe. Nurses working with Project Enhance confided that by witnessing the astounding progress their participants have demonstrated, the nurses themselves are inspired to make improvements to their own lives. Nurses praised the way Project Enhance focuses on empowering participants to take charge of their lives and discover ways to improve their lifestyle rather than simply telling participants what they need to do. A Chinese proverb says, "Give a man a fish and you will feed him for a day; teach a man to fish and you will feed him for a lifetime." Project Enhance is about teaching the elderly to "fish" for the ways to improve their quality of life.

NOTE: This paper was written while the author was an intern with the Coordinating Center of the Centers for Disease Control and Prevention-Healthy Aging Research Network (CDC-HAN) at the University of Washington and Senior Services in Seattle, Washington.

EBP Pearl

Evidence-based programs and interventions change lives—of patients and providers!

The Spirit Is Moving: How Evidence-Based Practice Can Impact Management Style

–Ellesha McCray, MSN, RN, MBA NE-BC
Nurse Manager
Veteran Affairs Pittsburgh Healthcare System, Pittsburgh, Pennsylvania

Evidence-based practice (EBP) has provided a framework for my administrative practice in various roles at the VA Pittsburgh Healthcare System (VAPHS). In my multiple roles within the VAPHS, evidence has been at the core of my administrative and clinical decision-making. The model of EBP that best describes my clinical and administrative practice is the Iowa Model. Utilizing this model, I have been successful at assessing the topic or problem, gathering the latest evidence related to the topic, and appraising the evidence. After research (or external evidence) has been reviewed, I pilot the change in practice. To facilitate a successful pilot, I select desired outcomes, collect baseline data, design EBP guidelines, and implement them. The next steps include evaluating the process and outcomes and modifying the practice guidelines as needed.

My experience with EBP at the program level began when I was the team leader for the Toyota Project. With this initiative, I reviewed infection control data, research, and staff practice data (internal evidence) to identify gaps or opportunities for improvement. At that time, sufficient evidence supported that adherence to CDC infection control guidelines would result in a reduction of hospital-acquired MRSA infections. Also, sufficient evidence from the automotive industry indicated that high quality could be achieved utilizing principles of the Toyota Manufacturing Company. Initially, our team established a goal or expected outcome of reducing hospital-acquired MRSA infections by 50% at the VAPHS. To achieve this goal, the Toyota Principles indicated that we need to standardize many of our processes to achieve the desired outcome. In addition, these principles supported engaging the staff who does the work, understanding that they have the insight as to how the work could be improved. Initially, I was very nervous and unsure of my team's ability to meet our goal. Still, trusting that these principles had worked for Toyota, we continued on our journey.

The Toyota model also supported use of the scientific method to guide change. It required staff to understand the current condition, to utilize epidemiological research and internal evidence to develop a target condition, and to clearly identify steps or interventions that will lead to the target conditions while monitoring or having a metric or built-in test to see if the target condition is working. Embracing and utilizing these principles were to result in quality outcomes for the patients in the form of safe and efficient care, staff engagement, and staff empowerment. Engaging and empowering staff to identify and resolve barriers to obtain improved patient outcomes was a difficult task. Yet helping staff nurses recognize the power of their insight was invigorating.

Small successes yielded more confidence for staff to tackle larger issues, which resulted in widespread success. It also instilled a sense of pride in the staff who were working in this area, which led to further engagement on the unit and development of the skill necessary to guide subsequent unit-based improvement. This method yielded positive results in our department. For example, our unit rate of hospital-associated MRSA infections decreased from 1.56 infections per 1,000 patient days to 0.63 infections per 1,000 patient days. We were very excited by this 60% reduction and extremely motivated to share our experience and spread our success. Later, we published our work in a peer-reviewed journal. Successfully implementing EBP was exciting, and it was personally satisfying to know that our efforts improved the lives of many patients by preventing infections. To have our work published for all to see and learn from was a highlight of my career and professionally satisfying. It is my hope that lessons learned through our experience will improve outcomes for many patients throughout the world.

To spread our success to the hospital, we again turned to the evidence to seek out an appropriate method. Research evidence showed that allowing staff to observe the success of one unit would provide a basis for them to improve their practice on their unit. After we implemented this plan, infection control practice across VAPHS improved, which contributed to a reduction in the incidence of hospital-acquired MRSA infections and other improved patient outcomes.

Moving to a new nurse manager position and away from team leading in the Toyota Project, I had lots of questions on leadership style, approach, and staff satisfaction. My new staff was not eagerly awaiting a new manager, so I was challenged to lead this group of clinicians with varying degrees of experience, a wide variety of personalities, and a reputation for being a very reactive unit. I was excited about this new opportunity, but I was nervous about the challenge. To prepare myself for these new challenges, I searched to find information about management styles and behaviors of an effective leader and a healthy work environment. The literature describes a healthy work environment as a work setting in which policies, procedures, and systems are designed so that employees can meet organizational objectives and achieve personal satisfaction in their work. Authors who publish in this area strongly suggest that authentic leadership is a key element to sustaining a healthy work environment. A healthy work environment supports communication and collaboration. This was the type of work environment that I wanted to build, so I began working to develop myself and my team toward that goal. Upon further review of the evidence, I found that managers who had shared governance structures reported higher job satisfaction, more effective decisions, increased staff accountability, and positive patient outcomes. In addition, shared decision-making or staff having the insight to change their work was a founding principle of the success of the Toyota Industry. I developed and implemented a shared decision-making structure on my unit. I role-modeled the new behavior I expected by leading by example, coaching, and mentoring staff toward the desired result.

Because EBP was the foundation of my practice, I modeled that evidence-based decision-making to encourage the staff to adopt that form of decision-making, which they did. For example, our professional practice council formulated fully documented evidence-based changes, such as requesting medications be added to their list of approved medications for their work area, standardizing handoff communication, reducing falls, reducing pressure ulcers, improving teamwork through visual communication tools, and shifting to a minimal lift culture. Over the past several years, EBP has enabled me to develop a highly functioning healthy work environment where staff nurses are proactive in taking on projects to improve our nursing unit. For example, greater than 50% of my registered nurses are involved in unit-based and/or hospital-wide projects or committees. Furthermore, our registered nurses indicated that they were highly satisfied with their work over the past few years, and patient satisfaction scores are consistently high. EBP has been the foundation for my nursing practice, no matter what my role, and will continue to guide my practice in the future.

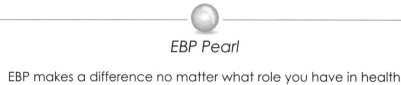

EBP Pearl

EBP makes a difference no matter what role you have in health care!

Chemotherapy Nurses: Improving Care From the Front Line

–Ellesha McCray, MSN, RN, MBA NE-BC, Nurse Manager

–Rayuana Zellars, MSN, RN-BC, Charge Nurse

Veterans Affairs Pittsburgh Healthcare System, Pittsburgh, Pennsylvania

On a routine day during my tour of duty, one chemotherapy patient, who we will call Rudy, at the Veterans Affairs Pittsburgh Healthcare System (VAPHS) was receiving Rituximab for the treatment of non-Hodgkin's B-cell lymphoma and began to experience rigors. Rigors are an adverse reaction that can occur in patients who are receiving a Rituximab infusion. According to the *American Heritage Medical Dictionary* (2007), rigors are defined as shivering or trembling, like when one has a chill, and can lead to a situation where organs or tissues have a decreased response to stimuli. Uncontrolled shaking and respiratory distress are two events that can accompany an episode of rigors. For Rudy, nursing staff immediately called a medical emergency code and waited for the physician to respond. While waiting for the physicians to come and treat the patient, I felt helpless because I could not provide any relief or comfort to Rudy, even though I knew the gold-standard treatment that should be provided for this condition. The physician team arrived within minutes, but it seemed like hours as we monitored the patient's condition. The physician gave Rudy a dose of Demerol in his intravenous (IV) line, which was effective for treating his rigors.

I discussed this situation with my colleagues and several of them had experienced the same thing. They also expressed a feeling of powerless as they waited for physician intervention when other patients experienced similar reactions to chemotherapy. After our discussion, a change in our nursing practice seemed imperative. I brought the issue to our unit-based Professional Practice Council (PPC) to discuss the feasibility and safety of chemotherapy-trained registered nurses (RNs) administering Demerol as a first-line therapy for patients experiencing rigors. My proposal included the RN being a first-line provider in managing rigors, instead of calling a medical emergency code. Initially, I reviewed evidence, appraised research, consulted oncology experts, and reviewed institutional policy regarding my plan for practice change. The path for introducing the evidence-based practice change involved our unit-based PPC, our institutional Clinical Leadership Council (CLC), and the support of our Nurse Administrative Leadership Council (NALC). After a series of approvals, our practice was expanded to include the administration of IV Demerol for patients experiencing rigors.

Rudy returned for another cycle of Rituximab. Once again, he experienced rigors. This time, nursing staff could administer IV Demerol right away, and the patient experienced immediate relief. It felt good to provide comfort to Rudy. I also felt empowered to manage to quickly relieve his distress. Rudy's response was most rewarding: "You girls really took care of that!"

Since the practice/policy change, chemotherapy-trained RNs act as first-line responders for chemotherapy patients experiencing rigors. Today, our process for intervening with rigors is more efficient and safe. In addition, care delays are decreased, response time is minimal, and the quality of care that chemotherapy nurses provide on my nursing unit has improved. Our practice change supports nursing autonomy and shared governance. We are proud of our staff and the meaningful contribution they have made towards positive patient outcomes.

As a nurse manager, it was frustrating to continually console my nursing staff as they raised care delay concerns with no plan for improvement. Improvement suggestions used to begin with phrases such as "Can't the physicians do something about this?" or "Someone should fix this." After reviewing the evidence on shared governance, I felt confident that my nursing staff could solve these patient care problems. My staff embraced the concept of shared governance and their power was unleashed. This was their first accomplished practice change, and it gave them the motivation to continue improvement initiatives that promote positive patient outcomes. Evidence-based practice laid the foundation for my nursing staff's autonomy in changing their practice and will be the central aspect of future improvements to their practice.

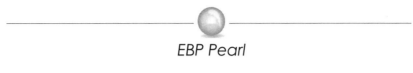

EBP Pearl

Never accept the status quo. Keep questioning—answers are there; you just have to look for them!

A Health Care Referral Process for the Homeless: Changing Lives

–Beth C. Norton, DNP, RN
Fort Walton Beach, Florida

A man named Clint was the inspiration for an evidence-based project to develop a health care referral process where none existed for use at a mission that housed homeless individuals. Clients who had medical or mental health illnesses and stayed at a local shelter for the homeless either were sent to the emergency department at a local hospital or the illnesses were ignored. Thirty-eight year old Clint was living in a meager house, worked almost every day, and was barely able pay his bills. He did not have health insurance, and this put him at risk for poor health. Clint, however, considered himself healthy, and he did not believe he needed preventative health care. Several of his teeth began to ache. He assumed he had some cavities, but he could not afford dental care. He became short-tempered and eventually lost his job and his home because of angry outbursts. He went to a local mission to live.

Clint said he was angry and that he was tired of not being treated fairly at the mission. He felt he was entitled to better treatment. By now, his mouth caused him continuous pain, he had an ear infection that did not respond to treatment, he was hard of hearing, and he had an ulcer on his leg that would not heal. As days turned into months, the mission staff and Clint missed at least one opportunity for free dental care that was offered through donations from a local church. It would be 8 months before the problem was resolved by the extraction of all his teeth, which were infected beyond repair. He was fitted with dentures, his hearing improved, and the continuous ear infections finally cleared up. Clint even noticed the infection on his leg finally began to heal. He realized how much pain he had been enduring from his infected mouth after the source of the pain was removed. His whole attitude about life changed for the better. Clint smiled more and was angry less. When asked what started the process of his turnaround, he said it was the people who just kept on caring about him even when he was rude to them and generally angry at the world. Homeless individuals tend to focus on immediate needs, leaving health problems to be addressed only when they become catastrophic.

The evidence-based project Clint inspired resulted in six protocols that outlined referral information to homeless mission personnel without using complicated medical jargon. The protocols are available online for any shelter, homeless mission, or halfway house to use at http://www.nhchc.org/tools.html. Local soup kitchens have introduced them to their volunteer staff so the volunteers can appropriately refer homeless individuals for the care they need.

Recently, a 47-year-old man named Ted took up residence at the mission where the protocols were used. Ted looked 10 years older than he stated and admitted that he was fighting a long-time addiction to cocaine. He had been clean and sober for 3 years when he started using cocaine again. He said that it did not take much for him to return to his old addiction, just a beer or two and he was on his way back to his "old friend" cocaine. He said the courts took away his son because of his addiction and that he lost absolutely everything that was once dear to him. When he came to the mission, he immediately joined the addiction recovery program and made plans to get his life back on track.

The mission was described as a "working mission," and Ted was assigned a job of helping to keep the mission clean. Ted was glad to work and stay busy; he said it kept him out of trouble. He was doing well until one day his head started hurting so bad that he had to lie down for a while. He told someone that in the past he had hypertension, but that his addiction took precedence over addressing the hypertension. It was discovered that Ted's blood pressure was 210/112, and he was sent to the emergency department at a local hospital since the protocol called for that immediate action. While there, Ted told the doctor that he had to urinate often, but that his urine volume was extremely low. The physician completed a prostate exam that Ted later described as the most painful exam he had ever experienced. Ted was given a prescription for an antibiotic to treat prostatitis. However, the exam was so painful and the infection so extensive that Ted could hardly walk the next day. The social worker at the mission talked with Ted and he asked to go back to work, but the pain from his prostate would cause him to have to return to his cot. The social worker followed the protocol to find a physician who would agree to see Ted. Eventually, a urologist agreed to see Ted at no cost and prescribed medication that resulted in great improvement. Two days later Ted was back on his feet, and his recovery from addiction continued. Ted was not sure what he would have done without the folks at the mission who cared enough and knew what to do to help him with the health problems he experienced. He smiled and said that after spending another month at the mission he will graduate from the recovery program and move into a job rehabilitation program. There he will progress through a more in-depth cocaine addiction recovery program and learn job skills to help him once again become a contributing member of his community. He had a sparkle in his eyes as he looked forward to the future.

The story does not end with Ted. Simply written for shelter volunteers who do not have a health care background, these evidence-based protocols are helping those who help the homeless to advise these individuals more appropriately. Homeless individuals who are helped by the protocols continue to tell their stories, which encourage shelter personnel to sustain the process.

NOTE: The names used in the story were changed, but the stories are true.

EBP Pearl

Everyone deserves evidence-based care!

My Journey

–Susan Schwerner, RN-ADN
Hudson Valley Hospital Center
Cortlandt Manor, New York

My journey began on my first day as an RN in 1992. I say this because nursing is just that, a journey. As a new nurse, I had great expectations of delivering the best care. Naive, maybe, but I was under the impression that nursing meant recognizing each patient as an individual while meeting their needs. To my dismay, as I progressed in my career, I began to realize that to meet all of the increasing demands of nursing, the focus of the nurse is more on the task than the patient. How quickly I lost my "new-nurse shine" as I focused on getting the job done to just survive and get through each shift. It became easier to accept the way care was delivered rather than to ask if there was a way to improve patient outcomes. As a result, I found myself reevaluating my role as a nurse.

After working many years in the same hospital, it became apparent that I needed a change. In December of 2006, I began a new job with hopes of renewing my spirit for nursing. After reevaluating my role as a nurse and finally making the long overdue change, I decided to approach nursing in a way that focused more on the patient than on the task. With a new job came new and different ways of delivering care. Little did I know of the great variances that occurred in clinical practice. With this realization, my journey would change to a positive new direction.

One thing that I have learned throughout my nursing career is to ask questions and not to assume anything. So when I was introduced to a new practice, the practice of administering IV push medications, I found myself asking many questions. Because this was a new practice for me, rather than assuming that I knew how to administer an IV push, I chose to ask what the proper procedure was at this hospital for administering an IV push medication. One medication in particular that I inquired about was Dilaudid because I observed patients having an adverse reaction immediately following administration. On one occasion, a patient stated that she would "rather deal with the pain than feel so sick; it makes me feel worse." After asking numerous RNs from different hospitals and different units, asking the pharmacy, and reading about Dilaudid, I began to realize that the protocol was very vague. The general answer was that it should be pushed slowly over 3–5 minutes. As to how to administer the medication, direction was vague. For example, I never received a satisfactory answer as to how to push a small dosage that may be equivalent to .5 cc over 3–5 minutes. With so many unanswered questions, I addressed my concerns to the Research Council in March of 2008.

With support from the Research Council, I began the disciplined evidence-based practice (EBP) process. First, I formulated a PICO (i.e., Patient population, Intervention or interest area, Comparison intervention or group, Outcome) question, which is a "focused clinical question." My patient population was inpatients receiving IV push medications. The intervention would be the safest and most effective method of administration. This would be compared with what I found to be variations in current practice. The outcomes I hoped to achieve were that the full dose would be received over a prescribed dosing period with minimal or no adverse reactions to improve patient satisfaction and outcomes.

Anecdotal evidence revealed that IV Dilaudid was a particularly problematic medication. A survey was then conducted among nursing professionals from various units on current practice to administer IV Dilaudid. The results of the survey showed variance in practice. The strategies most often employed by RNs were to dilute Dilaudid with saline push before administering; followed by a saline push, Dilaudid pushed undiluted; followed by a saline push and Dilaudid mixed with 50 cc NS to be given as a piggyback. Although these are all acceptable strategies, the consistency of duration of the "push" itself is difficult to determine without actual observation. Also, attention needs to be paid to fluid-restricted patients and the use of piggybacks. With this in mind, a new question arose: What is the standard to be?

Aware of the lack of clear direction from the literature, the hospital educators encouraged me to contact the pharmacy to obtain manufacturer guidelines. The manufacturer's recommendations for use of IV push medications included an instruction to administer these slowly, in some cases as low as 5 minutes, in others as high as 20 minutes. After seeing the results, I decided to search further. In January of 2009, I contacted two companies that distribute Dilaudid. Neither company gave me any more information besides to push it over 3–5 minutes. In my own experience, patients often experienced adverse reactions, such as dizziness, nausea, and sometimes vomiting with this rate of administration. Furthermore, both manufacturers agreed that the protocol was vague and did not include direction for dilution, nor did either offer any evidence base for their recommendations.

Upon researching the relationship between IV push and adverse events in the literature, I found little evidence to support an increased incidence of adverse reactions with the use of IV medications. I decided to do some internal investigation, so I contacted the pharmacy to find out how many adverse reactions to IV medications had been reported to the Adverse Drug Reaction (ADR) line and learned that there were none. Inquiring of the nursing staff, I learned that "nausea, vomiting, dizziness, and itching" with IV

Dilaudid was expected. In other words, the staff did not see these reactions as adverse events, but rather as normal sequelae of administering this drug. With the results of our research still leaving questions unanswered, we agreed that to ensure a standard of care, we must develop a protocol based on the evidence, patient preference, and clinician expertise (all key elements of EBP). However, first we needed the evidence to support a change in practice. With the help of the director of pharmacy, a form was developed for reporting ADRs in April 2009. Incentive was provided to nursing staff to report adverse events, and a representative of the pharmacy went to each unit weekly to remind staff to report these events. A flyer was developed as well to remind staff to report these adverse incidents. For 9 months, I collected and analyzed the data, which revealed that adverse reactions to IV push medications were indeed prevalent. In fact, we found they were three times more prevalent than to the same medication administered by IV piggyback medication. Patient safety, comfort, and satisfaction were compromised.

For the first time I felt that, as a nurse, I could create change that would improve care and enhance patient outcomes, comfort, and satisfaction. Eventually, we found research evidence that supported a change in practice. In 2010, the Institute for Safe Medication Practice (ISMP) recommended avoidance of the term "IV push" and recommended strategies to improve practice. Finally, after years of perseverance, dedication, and patience, I was able to develop a policy for "IV direct" medications that standardized the dilution and administration of IV narcotics and other frequently administered IV medications administered by RNs. The policy was reviewed by the Pharmacy and Therapeutics Committee, a committee of the Medical Board, and approved. We are now investigating the use of IV syringe pumps—such as those used in NICU—for the administration of "IV direct" medications to adults. We are working with the IT department and pharmacy to get specific directions for how these medications are to be administered put directly on the Medication Administration Record (MAR). Although more work needs to be done before this new policy becomes fully implemented, this experience has been very rewarding. It has reinforced that I have a greater role in patients' care that extends beyond the traditional tasks to which nurses have grown accustomed. I am energized to improve practice and reignited to make sure each patient receives the best possible care. By researching clinical issues that emerge at the bedside, nurses can utilize the knowledge generated to provide excellent care. Hopefully, through my experience, other RNs will feel empowered to improve care by recognizing that they can make a difference. At the bedside 24 hours a day, 7 days a week, nurses utilize their critical-thinking skills to keep patients safe, detect emerging problems, and save lives. Feeling as though my journey has gone full circle, I have been inspired to give a higher quality of personalized care by meeting the special needs of each patient. I joined both the Research Council and the Performance Improvement Council so that I can share my newly gained expertise.

NOTE: Special thanks goes to Chris Malmgreen, RN-BC, MA, MS, CHES

EBP Pearl

EBP change to improve patient outcomes often starts with one clinician's spirit of inquiry and persistence through the "character builders" to make a positive difference.

Putting Evidence-Based Knowledge Into Practice

–Linda J. Smith, BSN, RN
Chair, Clinical Practice Committee
Portland VA Medical Center, Portland, Oregon

The following story is just one out of dozens of examples of how Portland Veterans Administration Medical Center (PVAMC) nurses translate evidence into practice to improve outcomes for our patients. The Clinical Practice Committee (CPC) does routine evaluations of our homegrown nursing procedures to ensure that how we practice the art of nursing is backed with evidence or the science of nursing.

Our process includes asking clinical questions, searching the literature, critically appraising studies, benchmarking with our peers, looking for standards of practice organizations and consulting expert nurses. This is accomplished at a frequency from yearly up to every 3 years, depending on the nature of the specific procedure. Approximately 7 months before a procedure is due to have the review completed, the chair of the CPC receives notice via a report from our own unique access database. The chair then asks the committee membership for a volunteer who has a particular interest in the procedure. Alternately, a content expert nurse from elsewhere in the organization may be asked to spearhead the review. The process of evaluation then proceeds until the reviewer has a draft developed to present to the CPC membership for approval. Often, the membership and the reviewer conduct several rounds back and forth between them as questions are asked and revisions are requested. After the CPC gives final approval, the procedure is placed on our intranet site for all to reference.

One such example is the procedure for therapeutic phlebotomy. This procedure was taken on by Lynette Figg, BSN, RN, CCRN. Lynette is not a member of the CPC. She is a nurse working in the Portland Outpatient Surgery and Procedure (POPS) Unit. She is a content expert who performs therapeutic phlebotomy. In the process of conducting her literature search, Lynette discovered two differences between what the evidence showed as best practice and what our facility was currently practicing.

One difference was the use of a blood pressure cuff and manometer to compress the arm versus the use of a disposable tourniquet. The evidence indicated that with the tourniquet, nurses had no effective way of knowing how tightly they were applying it to the patient's arm. It could be applied looser than recommended or, conversely, too tightly, risking harm to the patient. The evidence went on to explain how to perform this procedure using a manual blood pressure cuff where the manometer can be watched so nurses can apply the specifically recommended amount of pressure consistently every time.

The second difference related to the way the tubing was disconnected when the procedure ended. The practice was to clamp the blood-filled tubing with a rubber band and then cut it with scissors. This approach allowed blood to splatter and drip. The evidence revealed a clamping device designed for this procedure existed that allowed for the safe clamping and cutting of the tubing without exposure to blood.

Lynette proposed that the procedure be changed to reflect these findings, which would require a practice change in her unit. An early discovery was that the POPS unit used primarily electronic blood pressure cuffs, which could not hold a partial pressure of 40mmHg as needed. They had only one manual cuff for emergency backup. To institute this practice change, they would need to secure more manual cuffs. Additionally, the unit would have to obtain the clamping devices. The unit clinical manager, Michael Fladland, was then consulted. Michael contacted supply processing and distribution and negotiated increasing the supply of manual blood pressure cuffs for the POPS unit. Michael then worked through proper channels with commodities and supply to purchase and stock the needed clamps in the POPS unit.

The procedure was approved by the CPC and posted to the website. Michael and the charge nurse, Den Ehrman, completed the necessary training of the POPS staff. Additional training is ongoing as new staff come on board to ensure that every nurse who is trained in performing therapeutic phlebotomy employs these safety devices with knowledge and competence.

The outcome is that our patients are now receiving the safest possible care during this procedure, and nurses have the satisfaction of knowing that they are providing that care. The risk of harm from a tourniquet applied too tightly for the 40-minute duration this procedure takes, or of exposure to splattered blood, has been eliminated.

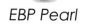

EBP Pearl

A process for regularly reviewing the evidence behind policies and procedures improves outcomes for patients.

Living Fit—One Step at a Time

–Karen Gabel Speroni, BSN, MHSA, PhD, RN
Director, Nursing Research and Chair, Research Council
Inova Loudoun Hospital and Inova Fair Oaks Hospital, Leesburg, Virginia

During my frequent international travel for drug and device development for treatment of osteoarthritis, my anecdotal data collection began on lifestyle and body-size differences between Americans and non-Americans. Most intriguing was the mounting evidence linking obesity with the development of subsequent comorbidities, yet Americans weren't sufficiently finding the balance between foods food and activity choices to avoid, succumbing to the pipeline of new drugs and devices to treat their obesity-related comorbidities. Though the need for nonpharmacological programs on healthy lifestyles was overwhelmingly clear, a gross shortage of these types of programs prevailed.

Years later when I became the Director of Nursing Research at Loudoun Hospital (now Inova Loudoun Hospital) in Leesburg, Virginia, I was asked by a visionary Chief Nurse Officer, Joy Solomita, to conduct a childhood obesity study to help children lose weight in the community our hospital served. At that time, Virginia was one of the unhealthier states with respect to obesity. Overweight status among American children ages 2–19 years was approximately 17%.

After pondering how I, as a nurse, might help children lose weight, the answer hit me as I was stepping on a cross-trainer at the gym, listening to another person who had the same aspirations. Pana DeGooyer, Good Sports Fitness, LLC, Leesburg, Virginia, and I quickly surmised we shared a passion for children to live fit in our community. Pana had created the Kids Living Fit exercise program. I developed the Kids Living Fit (KLF) research study program. The program included Pana's KLF exercise component, yoga, and the hospital components, which were development and support of the research requirements and methodologies. In addition to the exercise and yoga, the research included registered dietitian (RD) sessions; weights and measures by registered nurses (RN) for body mass index (BMI) percentiles, adjusted for age (months) and gender; and creation of diaries to raise awareness in child-study participants regarding the balance between daily foods consumed and activities chosen.

At the time of the research development in 2004–2005, the literature lacked studies about the effect of school- or hospital-based programs on both preventing overweight status among normal weight children and reversing unhealthy BMI status among overweight children. I worked with fellow RNs, RDs, statisticians, exercise trainers, and yoga teachers to design and test, over a series of three studies, whether the KLF intervention could make a positive impact in children's BMI percentiles when implemented as an afterschool or hospital-based program. The objective of the KLF studies was to provide school- and community-based programs that enhanced the health of elementary-school-aged-children. We predicted that the KLF group would have a decrease in their average BMI percentile after participating in the KLF intervention.

Two pilots and one larger comparative project comprised the three KLF studies. The school-based studies, for second to fifth graders of all BMIs, were one pilot (N=14) and one comparative (N=194, Intervention group=86, and Contrast group=108). The hospital-based study (N=32) included children 8–12 years of age with a BMI of greater than or equal to the 85th percentile. The studies were a series of 8–12 weekly sessions and exposed children to a variety of physical activities that could subsequently be pursued independently. All programs included teaching healthy lifestyle choices of best choice foods and demonstration and teaching of active behaviors. The RDs presented nutrition information, including portion distortion and best food choices. We worked with the county school RDs to determine the best option for children to choose from the school menus during the weeks the research was ongoing. We encouraged children to select what was *Best4u* versus what they wanted. School lunch menus were tagged with *Best4u* choices. Menus also were created for bringing lunches from home. Parental attendance was encouraged for the RD lectures. Nurses conducted pre- and post-measures for BMI and waist circumference. Participants completed study diaries documenting pedometer totals, daily activities (sedentary and nonsedentary), and foods consumed, including fast-food meals and best choice meals. Results of the three studies demonstrated decreases in age-adjusted BMI and waist circumference and increases in physical activity.

We published our three research studies and also disseminated our study findings through podium presentations and poster presentations at local, national, and international meetings. The research was profiled as an Agency for Health Care Research and Quality innovation. We also were asked to present to our county school board to provide recommendations for decreasing obesity in the children in our schools. Recommendations included having the school nurse or clinic's aide obtain each child's BMI percentile, adjusted for age (months) and gender, at the beginning of the year and providing this confidential information to the parent, along with an interpretation of the percentile. All parents also would be provided information on services in the community that could be utilized for children at risk of becoming overweight or who were overweight.

As the prevalence of childhood obesity continues to increase at alarming rates, more patients are going to require nursing care for chronic comorbidities. We must offer programs that focus on healthy weight management and obesity. Inova Fair Oaks Hospital, one of the two hospital-based KLF pilot study sites, utilized the evidence from the study as part of the foundation to create two childhood obesity programs, FUN (Fitness &

Understanding Nutrition) and SNAP (Simple Nutrition and Physical Activity). These hospital-based obesity programs do focus on healthy weight management and obesity prevention for children ages 7–15 years.

Nurses can take the initiative to implement programs using the evidence in the published literature, including the KLF research, to offer hospital and/or school-based programs to educate children, including those who are overweight (or at risk for becoming overweight), and to teach healthy lifestyle choices regarding exercise, activities, and nutrition.

The need for programs for adults prevails, with an estimated obesity rate for American adults of 65%. Nurses on the forefront of patient care have a distinct opportunity to educate patients about healthy lifestyle choices regarding exercise, activities, and nutrition. They also have the same healthy lifestyle education opportunities with their families and those they interact with in their communities.

Our next step to decrease obesity was taken in 2009 when the Nurses Living Fit (NLF) study was developed after the KLF model. The literature did not reveal programs for nurses to live healthier lifestyles. In 2010, we began the prospective, quasiexperimental, multicenter, hospital-based NLF research study at seven hospitals in three states. The NLF intervention included 12 weekly sessions of once-weekly exercise, once-monthly yoga, and once-monthly nutrition education lectures. The hypothesis tested was that the NLF intervention group would experience a significantly greater mean BMI reduction compared to the contrast group not participating in the intervention. The objective of this study was to quantify the change in BMI pre- and post-measures between the NLF and contrast groups. Participants in the NLF intervention group were all nurses who underwent a 12-week program including weekly exercise sessions, monthly yoga sessions, and monthly nutrition lectures by RDs. The NLF group participants completed study diaries during the intervention period (Weeks 1, 4, 8, 12) and at the final study follow-up time period (Week 24). Both groups had BMI and waist measures at Baseline, Week 12, and Week 24.

Preliminary NLF results in this ongoing research demonstrate a decrease in BMI and/or waist circumference for the NLF group. The majority of participants indicated they would recommend the NLF program to other nurses and health care employees.

It is important for health care organizations to offer evidence-based programs that educate nurses/employees on balancing exercise and nutrition to achieve and maintain normal weight. Hospitals can use the evidence from the NLF research model to provide evidence-based programs to facilitate education of their nurses on healthy lifestyle principles incorporating the balance between exercise and nutrition. Ideally, nurses can utilize these principles to achieve and/or maintain normal weight and to better educate their patients, their families, and communities, on healthy lifestyle principles targeting healthy weight management and obesity prevention.

We continue to take one step at a time at Inova Loudoun Hospital to improve the health of our patients and community, including our employees. Our next step is to offer "Health Care Employees Living Fit." When we initiated the NLF study, we had requests from non-nurses, including physicians, to participate in the NLF program. Other hospitals have asked if they can initiate the program.

To offset the associated labor costs and other direct costs of these programs, the Research Council holds an Annual Nurses Living Fit 1 mile/5k Walk/Run event. Funds received from these events support nursing research. The Office of Women's Health provided a grant in 2010 for Women's Health Week to support this event.

Take the initiative to develop a healthy lifestyle program in your hospital or school, targeted for the group most in need in your community, whether children or adults, nurses or doctors. Living fit takes one step at a time!

EBP Pearl

Research conducted, but not put into practice, will have no benefit for patients and communities; we must move evidence from research into practice to improve health outcomes.

Should Constipation Be the Sixth Vital Sign?

–Tamara Ventura, BSN, RN, OCN
Virginia Goff, BSN, RN, OCN
Providence St. Peter Hospital, Olympia, Washington

Constipation is such a basic, "Nursing 101" topic that we thought that after 20 years of nursing we couldn't learn anything else about it—until we examined our own patient statistics. Many times, because of competing priorities, constipation prevention has become an afterthought rather than treated with a proactive approach. The delay in preventing and treating constipation results in a longer length of stay and increases costs. In addition, it allows for a negative impact on the quality of life of our patients. As experienced registered nurses, we returned to school for our BSN degrees to improve our practice and patient outcomes. During our Introduction to Research class, we discovered that it takes approximately 17 years for evidence to make it to the bedside. We were shocked. We were given examples of how many things we do on a daily basis that are not rooted in the best evidence, but done through tradition, because that is the way we've always done it. Since then, our eyes were opened to look at our practice in a different fashion and to question our practice, looking for the best way to deliver care to our patients. Only through analyzing everyday bedside nursing care, comparing it to the available evidence in the literature, and making any necessary changes can nurses be sure they are providing their patients with the very best in quality care. After making any changes, nurses are encouraged to complete the nursing process by evaluating the effectiveness of any modifications made.

Constipation, a nurse-driven outcome, was a subject at the Institute of Learning conference sponsored by the Oncology Nursing Society in 2006. Initially, it did nothing to excite us, until the speaker shared the exorbitant cost involved in its treatment and the extended length of stay that results from this problem. We found that, annually, billions of dollars are spent evaluating and treating all patients with constipation, with direct medical costs in the millions. We became inquisitive about how these results of constipation would compare to our practice setting in the acute care hospital and started our journey of discovery. Since we work with oncology patients, we wanted to make a difference to that population and decided to look at opioid-induced constipation in adults as that would include most inpatients.

Nurses still acknowledge the importance of constipation prevention, but somehow in our bustling priority index, it falls short in significance. However, for the patient taking opioids, constipation continues high on the list of essential acute symptom management and affects their quality of life. A couple of examples that we have encountered in our practice include:

- K.S., a 20 year old who had recently gone through a tonsillectomy, was given Codeine elixir for pain control. She was being admitted for abdominal pain, which turned out to be caused by constipation, and needed "enemas till clear." This patient was totally mortified. She was never told to monitor her bowel habits while taking the Codeine, and being so young, she wasn't in the habit of doing so. Among the oncology population, opioid-induced constipation is a universal problem. We have seen patients admitted with nausea and vomiting and partial bowel obstructions because of opioid-induced constipation that was ill-managed at home.

- J.G. was a 68-year-old patient admitted for dyspnea and pain related to his lung cancer. He received chemotherapy and was placed on hydromorphone through a patient-controlled anesthesia (PCA) machine while in the hospital. On day five of his hospitalization, he was due to be discharged when he informed the physician, "I haven't moved my bowels since I've been here." His discharge was delayed and Lactulose was started until his constipation was resolved, adding 2 days to his length of stay (LOS).

Currently, in many situations, constipation is primarily treated retrospectively and undermanaged at best, thus, in many cases producing a delay in discharge.

Research states prevention of constipation is the preferred treatment. We evaluated our current practice and found areas for improvement. Statistics from our 350-bed hospital revealed 723 adult patients were admitted from October 2007 through October 2008 with a diagnosis of constipation. The average LOS for these patients was 6.7 days, which represents 2 days longer than our hospital's average LOS for the acute patients. We estimated that by decreasing our LOS those 2 days by proactively preventing and treating constipation as an early intervention, our hospital can save approximately $1,800.00 per case, and $1,301,400.00 per annum.

Based on our synthesis of the available data and the importance of continually assessing our practice toward an evidence-based quality approach, we concluded that it was imperative that we adopt a proactive method in preventing constipation and utilize an early intervention process in treating this symptom. We examined our processes and focused on education. Others needed to be aware of the benefits available to the patient and the hospital by preventing this common side effect. We thought, "Constipation should be the sixth vital sign." Adding this easy intervention would assist the nurses in improving the monitoring of constipation, which is the first step of prevention. Utilizing the evidence in the literature, we created an algorithm of a simple bowel regimen and a table for review of Categories of Laxatives and their Mode of Action as a tool for our nurses and posted it on our in-house nursing website. Our recommendation was that our hospital add a stool softener and stimulant laxative alternative on the preprinted patient-controlled anesthesia (PCA) forms to prevent constipation in patients receiving opioid therapy through this route.

We have disseminated education to the hospital nursing staff through two different avenues to heighten awareness of the underassessment and under treatment of constipation and the need for a proactive approach in prevention of this problem. We have prepared an educational poster and presented it at our hospital's Nursing Congress Forum and displayed it through the nursing education department in the cafeteria. In addition, we have written a short article of the same content in our in-house weekly publication, *Nursing Notes*, and plan to present further education on "the sixth vital sign" at selected staff meetings. After the education process is completed, we plan to follow up with an additional query to verify the improvement that we have made. This follow-up will improve the quality of our patient care through evidence-based nursing, increase our patient's quality of life, and reduce costs through indirect and direct measures by decreasing the patient's length of stay associated with undertreatment of the common side effect.

You may discover that your facility is not an exception to the literature, having an extended length of stay and incurring an increase in costs because of this basic problem. Even though constipation is a Nursing 101 problem, we can make a difference for the patient and the hospital by adopting it as the sixth vital sign.

EBP Pearl

Whenever possible, clinicians need to measure both patient outcomes and costs saved with the implementation of evidence-based practices.

IVs and Evidence-Based Practice in the Emergency Room

–*Rosalyn Webb, BSN, RN*
Program Manager, Digestive Diseases
Maine Medical Center, Portland, Maine

My first lesson with research and evidence-based practice (EBP) was a few years into my nursing career. The first years were focused solely on honing nursing skills and assessment and laying the foundation of my nursing practice so I could expand and start to think critically about my patients. As soon as I made the leap from novice to experienced emergency department (ED) nurse, I began to see processes and practices differently, opening the door for EBP.

One of these practices in the emergency department was to remove any IV started in the prehospital setting and replace the IV with a new one in the ED for all patients being admitted, even with no signs of infection, infiltration, redness, palpable cords, pain for the patient, or difficulty flushing the line. This made little sense to me, and I knew it was not an experience that enhanced patient satisfaction. I finally asked why we did this, because IVs started within the hospital walls without any of complications could stay in a patient 72 hours! "That's the way it's done," was the response I received. The policy backing this was over 10 years old.

Because I was not content with that response, I dug into the research on the topic. I found that a few clinical trials had been done to track infection and complication rates of peripheral lines started in the prehospital setting versus the hospital setting. However, I found a large body of research concerning hospital infection rates in peripheral lines.

The common theme in all the research in pre-hospital and in the acute hospital settings was the preparation of the site *before* the line entered the vein.

After speaking with my nurse manager about the issue, I found myself in front of the hospital infectious disease committee with my research in tote. I was nervous, having never done anything like this before! I proposed a change in the decade-plus-old hospital policy requiring all prehospital peripheral IVs to be removed automatically. My proposal would allow the professional RN to assess the need for an IV change and to watch for signs of infection/complications. I shared the research. I also discussed the business case for the proposed change by highlighting the cost savings with a reduction of IV catheters, heparin locks, and IV start kits utilized and the valuable RN time that could be better used providing a different patient service. The most important factor was one of patient satisfaction, which would rise as patients would be happier with less IV sticks, less discomfort, and fewer breaks in their skin for potential microbes to enter to cause infection.

Committee members had many questions regarding my suggested practice change, which had not been changed in so many years, based on a fear that peripheral lines started by EMTs and paramedics in the field had higher infection rates. This information had come out of the first meeting. All of my answers were based on the evidence from research that I provided to them, not fear or assumptions. I did not attempt to create answers on my own; I let the data speak for itself.

The committee considered my proposal and wanted me to speak in front of the hospital nursing practice committee to explain my research and proposed practice change, which I did. I had even more research for that meeting; the CDC had just updated the guidelines for peripheral lines. It was hot off the press, and it backed my case.

After many months, I was successful in changing the hospital policy. IV lines started in a prehospital setting without signs of complications could be left in an admitted patient for 48 hours. I also successfully published a short review article in the *American Journal of Nursing* that discussed the research surrounding prehospital IV starts and how long the lines should be left in hospitalized patients.

This process was a wonderful educational experience for me. It was the first of many evidence-based platforms I have been involved in to better patient care. I also learned how to carefully and critically appraise the available research, examining how the studies were conducted, comparing results from one study to another, and considering the validity of results.

I am now a program manager at a different hospital and involved in data collection, program development, and patient safety and satisfaction, all of which I could not be successful at without evidence-based practice!

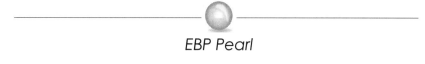

EBP Pearl

Data speak loudly; equip yourself with evidence in making practice change recommendations, and you will succeed!

Softening Patients' Comfort with Evidence-Based Practice

–Barbara A. Wolfe, RN
Staff/Charge Nurse, Emergency Department
MetroHealth Medical Center, Cleveland, Ohio

I am a 30-year part-time staff/charge nurse in our 90,000+ Level I Trauma Center Emergency Department (ED). I began my job as "Quiffer" (Quality Improvement Facilitator) for our ED in 2006. With this extra position, I found great satisfaction in studying and evaluating our own patient care delivery system and how various aspects of it could be improved.

In 2008, with all of the emphasis on evidence-based practice and the Centers for Medicare & Medicaid Services' (CMS) noncoverage of nosocomial occurrences, I began to research backboard usage and the practice of early removal of patients from the backboard. Backboards are used primarily by rescue squads for transporting patients to the hospital, but after the patient is in the emergency department (ED), they are often used as a means to keep patients flat and to aid in movement from one surface to another. This is not the intended use of the backboard. I found an abundance of literature citing the dangers of prolonged backboard immobilization, especially the increased development of pressure ulcers, decreased respiratory function, and decreased patient satisfaction. Also, many EDs across the country and in other countries had already adopted the practice of early removal of patients from backboards. Our department and hospital are deeply committed to constantly improving patient care and satisfaction; hence, my evidence-based performance improvement (PI) project was born.

I gathered evidence and sought the assistance of my ED clinical nurse specialist (CNS) and our ED Unit Practice Committee and began to plan my strategy. It began, as always, with problem identification. We identified several factors contributing to the length of time spent on backboards. Nurses lacked a process for independent backboard removal. They also lacked communication with physicians when removal was clearly indicated. A sudden influx of patients caused delays in radiographic study completion, and staff were not always available to log-roll patients off boards. Additionally, patients' cognitive impairments affected their ability to comprehend the need to remain lying flat.

After identifying contributing factors, we looked for ways to improve our process. The evidence in the literature cited specific criteria nurses could use to assess for early backboard removal. We used these as the basis for our PI project. We then wrote, got approval for, and initiated a policy for removing backboards from ED patients. The purpose of this was to give the nurse, under very specific guidelines, the ability to make the decision to remove the backboard without a physician order. This policy refers only to patients arriving in the main department that are not classified as "traumas." After the policy was approved, I sent paper copies of the policy, along with specific instructions to each staff member, posted flyers around the department, and verbally educated staff. This policy was rolled out in May 2009. I also encouraged removal of the board as early as safely possible for the "trauma" patients. These are patients that meet specific criteria and are treated in our trauma bays with a specific trauma team present, along with the ED staff. In many of the trauma cases, patients were first being stabilized in the ED, transported to CT scan and X-ray, then returned back to the ED, all while remaining on the backboard. This would usually take well over an hour, many times longer, depending on the number of traumas and extent of backup.

In my initial data collection, I did a retrospective chart review (random and only a percentage of the backboarded patients). This showed an average of 90 minutes spent on the backboard. I also did a real-time assessment of patients' level of comfort on and off the board, and, surprise, this study showed that the patients were much more comfortable off the board. Imagine that!

My goal was to decrease the average time by at least 30 minutes. During the first quarter (still doing random and percentage audits), our time was decreased dramatically to an average of 35 minutes on the board. By this time, I and many of my fellow staff had become fully inspired and jumped into this project with both feet, as they say. It was truly gratifying to see a patient care improvement initiative being adopted by the entire staff.

Thinking "well, my work here is done," I relaxed and prepared to let the project go into autopilot. Silly me. The second quarter times went back up to 59 minutes, for a 6-month average of 47 minutes—not as wonderful as I had hoped. What happened? In investigating the problem, I began tracking every trauma patient that arrived in our ED (approximately 350–450 per month)—no easy feat! I found that the backboard times varied from just a few minutes to 3 hours and more.

As I reviewed the outcome data, I discovered a few issues. Though anywhere from 350–450 patients per month arrived on backboards (and this is only the actual trauma patients), only about 40–45% were having their times documented in the ED record. In an effort to improve this number, I again went on an education campaign with the staff. With the help of my unit manager and nursing director, I also obtained a notation button placed in the electronic medical record (EMR) that specifically states "backboard removed," "spinal precautions maintained," or "cleared by . . ."

Another big issue that came to my attention was that the radiology department was uncomfortable with patients being removed from backboards while still being on spinal precautions. Our present practice was that if the patient was not on a board, they could be dropped off in radiology without our medic staying with them. Radiology was concerned that the patient would not be monitored for precautions, and if they were still in spinal precautions, the radiology techs would not necessarily be aware. We instituted "ticket to ride" forms that accompany patients, and if they are off the board and still on precautions, the medic stays with them in radiology. During this time, I had a discussion with our Trauma Program Coordinator, an RN who was very excited about this initiative, and expressed a desire to make this a house-wide effort. She told me that she received a request from radiology that we provide their techs with training on log-rolling patients that are not on a backboard. In the meantime, a new trauma surgeon who came from an institution that was already practicing early backboard removal arrived and began removing patients from the boards during the secondary survey. Now, everyone was up in arms. This suddenly became a huge issue, almost one year after its inception! Needless to say, I was thrilled.

Meetings between the ED, trauma, and radiology ensued. It was agreed that the entire hospital should "be on the same page," so to speak, about this issue. As we discussed issues such as radiology's insistence that it takes at least four people to "log-roll" a patient, so the ED should provide these four people, we realized that we had a semantics problem. During one of our meetings, we all went on a "field trip" to both the ED and X-ray department. We demonstrated the technique of using a slide board to move patients that are not on backboards, and X-ray showed us that, for plain TLS spine films, they needed the backboard to raise the patient up for better visualization of the spine. We came to an agreement that for those patients who need plain spine films (estimated to be about 15 per month), we would supply a board to be kept in radiology, and they would call for moving assistance that we would provide when needed.

Meetings have been ongoing, and we (ED, trauma, and I with the support of my unit manager, CNS, and nursing director) are remaining strong in our resolve to decrease patients' time on backboards. As of this writing, the times are decreasing, but we still have not come to a defined agreement for creation of a house-wide protocol.

I cannot begin to describe how much this project has inspired me. As a result, I have gone on to suggest and begin other evidence-based performance improvement projects and have become extremely involved in evaluating and putting together staff education to improve the quality of our ED nursing care. I am actually eligible to retire (a few months ago), but I feel I'm just not ready to give up not only my couple nights a week of patient care, but (and maybe even more importantly at this point) my newfound responsibilities of nursing improvement and inspiring my co-workers to move to the higher plane of the very best evidence-based care delivery possible.

EBP Pearl

Don't ever underestimate what just one passionate, dedicated person can do to improve the evidence-based care of patients!

The Evidence-Based Practice for Pressure Ulcers

–Mary Kathleen Wood, BSN, RN
Nurse Manager, Wound Center at South Miami Hospital

–Carolyn L. Lindgren, PhD, RN
Research Specialist, Baptist Health South Florida

–Mercedes M. Condom, BS, PCCN, RN
Assistant Nurse Manager, Step-down Unit, South Miami Hospital
South Miami, Florida

Pressure ulcers remain a major challenge for nurses in acute care. Prevention, early detection, assessment, and treatment of pressure ulcers require vigilant, organized care. The unrelenting problem of pressure ulcers is prominent in national health care forums' regulations, including the Institute for Healthcare Improvement (IHI) initiatives for patient safety, the Centers for Medicare & Medicaid Services (CMS) regulations on reimbursement to hospitals for patient care when a pressure ulcer is acquired in a health care institution, and the National Pressure Ulcer Advisory Panel (NPUAP) joining with the European Pressure Ulcer Advisory Panel (EPUAP) on consolidating guidelines for practice. For nurses, care of pressure ulcers is seen by some as a less interesting and unrewarding aspect of bedside care when compared to high technological interventions that yield positive patient outcomes that are more instantaneous.

At South Miami Hospital, a 160-bed acute care hospital, the Wound Center and Hospital Acquired Pressure Ulcer Group (HAPUG) undertook a highly focused and results-driven approach to reducing pressure ulcer incidence rates and aggressively treating patients with pressure ulcers. The approach took the problem from the bedside to research and back to bedside in a span of 2 years. The purpose of the evidence-based project was to develop up-to-date standards of care for prevention of pressure ulcers and treatment modalities for patients with pressure ulcers. The impact of the project has changed not only bedside care for our patients, but also has fortified the purpose and meaning of *high-touch nursing care.*

The evidence-based project started with gathering evidence. Review of the current literature included applicable research studies and guidelines of professional nursing care and governmental regulations. The gathered material was reviewed and sorted into two groups to identify what must occur at the bedside from a regulatory perspective, what care practices are supported by research, and what the standards of care are for pressure ulcers. The current clinical practices were documented by the Wound Center, rounding on patients on the various floors of the hospital. The current practices in the hospital were compared to the practice recommendations from the literature review. The findings from the review and the patient care observation data were presented to nursing leadership, and a charged discussion concerning the barriers nurses face to provide ideal care for patients with pressure ulcers resulted. The results were renewed vigor and dedication by all involved to make a workable, standardized plan for pressure ulcer prevention and treatment.

The salient points from the leadership discussion were noted, compiled, and addressed. Then an outline for the project was composed. A quick review of Lewin's Change Theory helped to organize the scope of the project in terms of driving and restraining forces and provided perspective on the complex nature of bringing about a change in practice and attitude in a complicated hospital system. The resistance to change described in Lewin's theory, and by Schein, who stated that "all forms of learning . . . start with some form of dissatisfaction . . . generated by data . . ." was observed in the nurses' responses to the proposed change in practice. The change would require effort and skill acquisition for the nurses. The steps of the project had to include garnering support from those nurses with resistance and appealing to their desire to provide excellent care.

A team of nurses dedicated to wound care existed but needed to be reorganized and to include support professionals. The newly organized wound team looked at specific processes in place that supported the goals of the project and identified needed changes.

These included adding pressure ulcer prevention education classes, promoting dialogue about pressure research findings among nurses, standardizing pressure ulcer prevention aides and products for nurses to choose from, and collecting current pressure ulcer incidence data on the nursing units. In addition, recognizing the need for improved communication between nursing and medical staff on pressure ulcer care and prevention was noted, especially because pressure ulcer care and identification had been viewed as primarily a nursing responsibility.

Implementing the new plan required anticipating some of the staff and physician reactions. The resultant plan included the following steps:

1. Collected data was presented to the staff and the physicians.

2. Current documentation of pressure ulcers was discussed.

3. Participatory bedside learning was promoted.

4. Government regulations were presented.

5. Explanation of how pressure ulcers impact patients and hospitals financially was presented to nursing staff.

6. How optimal care of pressure ulcers aligns with patient and family satisfaction goals also was presented.

Identifying what the new standards should look like and how to implement the change was the next step. The wound team knew that nursing and allied health always enjoy learning new or renewing old skills and that this would positively drive the change. The wound team also knew that the willingness for nursing and medical staff to participate in patient safety, support quality initiatives, and maintain fiscal stability had always been a constant.

The standardized practices have been instituted, and the resulting effect has been that nurses reawakened to the power that evidence-based care can produce outcomes that make a difference for the patients. Physicians have realized the importance of having a team of nurses knowledgeable of the impact of comorbidities on the skin. There are enhanced fields on electronic documentation screens, frequent interactive inquiry on documentation issues with the Wound Center team, and increased cross-communication among all members of patient care providers. An unexpected but welcomed benefit is that improvement in interactions has removed the hierarchical attitudes among physicians, nurses, and wound team leaders, and a collegial approach is evident.

The development of standardized care for pressure ulcers and the education and dissemination of those findings has resulted in improved care of patients with potential pressure ulcers and those with ulcers. The operation and effectiveness of this improved evidence-based practice strategy is seen in one nurse's observations of pressure ulcer care on the step-down unit:

> *"I am currently the Assistant Nurse Manager for the step-down unit at SMH and a member of the HAPUG. In my unit, we have our share of highly complicated pressure ulcers. We currently have a patient that has been in our care for over 3 months. This particular patient, when admitted to our unit, had a stage four sacral ulcer. By implementing our EBP wound care set of orders and having our wound care team involved, this particular patient's decubitus improved in a way I never imagined. The stage four decubitus has improved to a stage two and still has the potential to heal . . ."* (Anonymous nurse, Step-down Unit, SMH).

In conclusion, the work has just begun, but using evidence-based practice principles has made a difference in the wound care at our hospital. Revising the new protocol as we observe the effect of the care now being provided and incorporating new research and practice knowledge is inevitable. The quest for better care to prevent and treat pressure ulcers is neverending, but improved care is possible.

EBP Pearl

Evidence-based practice not only improves patient outcomes, it also enhances a transdisciplinary collegial approach to practice.

5

Fostering Teamwork With Evidence-Based Practice

Individuals can accomplish much, but teams can accomplish more. Imagine what it would be like to sail by yourself in the America's Cup, a highly unique race with specially built yachts. These sleek vessels require an active 17-person crew to be in the race; to win, the crew has to be cohesive, proficient, and determined. Sounds like health care, doesn't it? For patients, providers, and systems to win, it is the team effort that will ensure success. The proficient team includes individuals who have shifted their paradigim to evidence-based practice (EBP) and are living that paradigm out in their daily decision-making, but it is coming together as a team that exponentially enhances their impact. The stories in this chapter are about fostering teamwork in EBP and how together these teams make a difference.

From the Heart: Improving Diabetes Care Through Evidence-Based Practice

–Mieca S. Valen, DNP, RN, CNP
Associate Professor, Winona State University
Rochester, Minnesota

Type 2 diabetes is nearly twice as prevalent in the Mexican-American Hispanic population as it is in non-Hispanic whites, and Hispanic persons are often diagnosed with diabetes at a later stage. My local community is no exception. Diabetes is the most frequently documented diagnosis among clients served at the local migrant health clinic where I am privileged to work as a volunteer nurse practitioner. The transient migrant lifestyle of many of our patients presents numerous challenges, including lack of re-sources, poverty, transportation difficulties, long work hours, and cultural and language barriers. Patients take time from their hectic work and life schedule to maneuver the challenges of the health care system only when they can no longer ignore symptoms of the disease. The high prevalence of Type 2 diabetes in our population inspires the mi-grant clinic staff to continually investigate ways to improve the health of this population.

Improvement in outcomes for Hispanic patients with type 2 diabetes was the goal of a nurse-led evidence-based project (EBP). Prior to development of the project, patients and staff at the migrant health clinic were interviewed to discover their perceived great-est need, and the approach to meeting this need that they thought would be the most effective. Overwhelmingly, those interviewed requested diabetes education, specifically related to nutrition and dietary management. High fat, high carbohydrate meals and snacks, including tortillas, refried beans, pork, and beef are common in this population. Patients, family, and staff reported that they wanted to learn how to incorporate their cultural favorites into a healthy diet. Staff reinforced the need for culturally appropriate patient education regarding nutritional management of Type 2 diabetes.

As I considered how to best meet these needs of our local population, I explored vari-ous ways of providing education to the Hispanic population. The majority of the popu-lation served at the clinic speaks Spanish and are members of either the local Hispanic residential or migrant communities. Community health workers (CHWs), as members of the community they serve, speak the language of the community, understand local community values, and incorporate cultural beliefs and practices into their work. CHWs can bridge gaps between people and resources and can integrate basic knowledge about disease prevention and care with local knowledge. Evidence supports that CHWs can efficiently and effectively deliver diabetes education, and in fact, CHWs have been shown to improve rates of diabetes education completion in Hispanic populations. As members of the Hispanic community, CHWs can provide diabetes education not only in the health care setting, but also on a daily basis as they interact with friends, family, and community members. Evidence also supports the benefit of cultural relevance in diabe-tes education. The desire to educate patients and families about diabetes and to improve their disease-related outcomes was at the root of this innovative, evidence-based educa-tional program developed and implemented by nurses and CHWs at the migrant health clinic.

An exciting aspect of this EBP was that from the initial stages, the project belonged to the entire team, especially the CHWs. Patients, family members, clinic staff, and providers all provided input into development of the project. Four bilingual health workers at the clinic served as CHWs and volunteered to participate in diabetes education training and to present the program to participants. They bought into the idea and worked hard to make the program successful, seeing the potential for improving the health of not only the participants of the program, but also the broader community. They also were willing to work hard and participate in nearly 30 hours of classroom education and planning, study on their own time, and complete a post-test following the training. As most of the CHWs did not have any formal education beyond high school and had full-time jobs and families to care for, this necessitated a considerable effort. There also was a certain amount of vulnerability required to venture into the unknown and learn the needed information. I was inspired by the enthusiasm shown by the CHWs and their willingness to give of their own time and energy to this project. After completion of the education, the CHWs were prepared to present the program to participants.

During the first session, which was presented entirely in Spanish by the CHWs, I had the realization that my work as project director was, for the most part, done. The CHWs presented the planned information, responded to questions, and interacted with the participants. They also prepared and shared a light meal of culturally relevant foods together, modeling appropriate portion sizes and carbohydrate choices. The confidence level of the CHWs increased tremendously through this experience. They were noted to ask more questions and seek out more learning during their regular work hours. The ability to provide accurate diabetes self-management education filled a need at the clinic. CHWs repeatedly indicated that they enjoyed the program and experienced increased satisfaction in their role at the clinic. They were able to use the information in the planned educational programs, in their daily work in the clinic, and in their community.

Implementation of this project was not without challenges. We had only three participants with diabetes who attended the entire series of six sessions, despite multiple recruitment methods. Numerous additional family members and patients with diabetes attended one or more sessions. Although the program required few health care resources, it did involve a considerable amount of CHW time. Because of the small number of participants, demonstrating a financial benefit of this program by measuring participant outcomes was difficult. CHW outcomes were largely anecdotal and difficult to measure. The literature included several well-designed research studies that provided evidence to support this project, but little information on its application to practice or appropriate outcome measures with such small participant numbers was available. This led to several key questions. How does one demonstrate the cost-effectiveness of a community-based educational program? What is an appropriate way to measure the community impact of CHW-delivered diabetes education? Perhaps more importantly, how can the benefit of the CHW to the community be measured?

Despite the challenges, however, this project improved the quality of the education available to our patients. In addition to the planned series of educational sessions, CHWs have been able to work with patients individually to provide diabetes education, thereby freeing up time for the providers and nurses to see more patients. They have also held numerous nutrition and physical activity classes at other events for patients with diabetes. The CHWs have the skills and materials needed to repeat the series of classes in the future. Most importantly, the CHWs can educate members of the Hispanic community about diabetes, perhaps leading to increased awareness of risk factors and earlier diagnosis. One CHW reported that she educated her child's daycare provider about diabetes. Another sought out additional information to share with his family, many who were living with Type 2 diabetes. A desired outcome of this increased awareness would be lifestyle changes that could decrease the incidence of Type 2 diabetes in the Hispanic community.

I experienced a great deal of personal satisfaction through the planning and implementation of this EBP. The prevalence of Type 2 diabetes and the late stage at which is often diagnosed in our patients is discouraging, and it is easy to become disillusioned. Prevention is a critical component in changing the current trend, yet we continue to see increasing rates of obesity and other risk factors for Type 2 diabetes in both our adult and adolescent population. Utilizing CHWs to educate the Hispanic population in both formal and informal settings could be one way to impact this trend.

I also grew in my leadership skills through implementation of this project. I learned that a key to successful leadership is involvement with and caring for the team. Each member of the team was valued and recognized. The combination of a cohesive team embracing the vision, research evidence supporting the project, and the team working together led to a successful evidence-based nursing intervention.

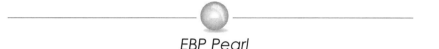

EBP Pearl

A caring leader who inspires confidence and conveys the vision of the project to the team has a greater chance of success.

Better Blood Pressure Measurement for Better Patient Care

–Kathleen A. Schell, PhD, RN
Interim Director and Associate Professor, School of Nursing
University of Delaware, Wilmington, Delaware

–Elisabeth Bradley, MS, APN, ACNS-BC
Clinical Leader Cardiovascular Prevention Program
Christiana Care Health System, Wilmington, Delaware

–Denise L. Lyons, MSN, GCNS-BC
Clinical Specialist in Gerontological Nursing, WISH Program Coordinator
Christiana Care Health System, Wilmington, Delaware

–Linda Bucher, PhD, RN, CEN
Professor, School of Nursing
University of Delaware, Wilmington, Delaware

–Maureen A. Seckel, MSN, APN, ACNS-BC, CCNS, CCRN
Clinical Nurse Specialist Medical/Pulmonary
Christiana Care Health System, Wilmington, Delaware

We were a team of nurses eager to begin our first clinical nursing research study. Our charge was to identify a research question relevant to a variety of practice settings in a major medical center. Our team represented critical care, medical-surgical, and maternity clinical specialties and included two staff nurses, a nurse manager, an informatics nurse, two educators, three clinical nurse specialists, and two school of nursing faculty. After several brainstorming meetings, the topic of increased use of the forearm for oscillometric blood pressures (BP) arose. Eyes widened and eyebrows rose in our meeting room. None of us had ever learned about or considered using that site for cuff placement, yet we had witnessed nursing assistants (nurse technicians) and direct care nurses doing so and with greater frequency. We were "on" to something!

Blood pressure measurement is a basic psychomotor skill learned during introductory nursing courses. Sphygmomanometers and automated/oscillometric machines are part of the routine equipment used in hospitals, home health care, clinics, occupational health offices, health screening events in malls, and many other settings. Subsequently, practicing nurses might deem BP measurement a mundane task, easily delegated, and one not requiring the expertise of a professional nurse. However, reflect on the implications of BP measurement: Should I administer this prescribed beta blocker medication to my patient? Should I allow my patient to sit in a chair today? Is my patient adequately hydrated? Could this elevated BP be the cause of my patient's headaches and/or an indication of a bigger problem? As you hopefully agree, the implications of the results of BP measurement are almost endless. Thus, accuracy of BP measurement is essential to provide appropriate health care. Overtreatment, inappropriate treatment, and even lack of treatment can result if an individual's BP is measured incorrectly. We agreed that BP measurement touched each of our clinical lives, those with whom we worked, but most importantly, our patients.

The American Heart Association's (AHA) gold standard of noninvasive BP measurement is the upper arm manual, auscultatory pressure. Automated oscillometric devices have grown in popularity because they are quick and convenient and eliminate some of the challenges of auscultatory technique. Circumstances such as arm size, available cuff sizes, and arm accessibility may prompt use of alternate sites such as the forearm, wrist, and calf. Yet variations in BP measurement are not always supported by expert opinion and/or research. Integration of best evidence to support institutional protocols on BP measurement is often lacking.

We were challenged to search and critically appraise scientific literature relevant to the use of the forearm for BP measurement. The hospital's librarians became our comrades as the research, practice, and educational literature in this area was difficult to find. Although forearm BPs were sometimes mentioned in manufacturers' and expert guidelines, references were not often provided in the sources. This scarcity of literature compelled us to conduct our first descriptive correlational study in 2003 with a convenience sample of 204 seated emergency department (ED) patients. Over the period of a year, we developed the research protocol, obtained IRB approval, and conducted data collector training. We were tuned into the AHA's recommendations for BP measurement. Using the ED setting was threatening to our group of novice investigators, but we sought a population of relatively healthy individuals with a wide age range. The ED provided a strong possibility of seeing a large volume of patients in a short time. We were individuals who had many other responsibilities, so we needed to be as efficient as possible during data collection. Working in pairs and using both of our hospital's ED sites, we managed to complete data collection in 3 weeks. We quickly coded and cleaned the data. We could barely wait for our statistician to share the results of our study. Ultimately, we found statistically significant differences indicating that forearm and upper arm BPs were not interchangeable when patients were seated with the forearm and upper arm placed at heart level.

We celebrated the completion of the study and shared our findings through presentations and a journal publication. However, we realized that our results, in addition to those results from one earlier investigation using noninvasive BP monitors, did not provide sufficient support to change practice. We needed to repeat our procedure in a different population and with subjects in different positions. Furthermore, we knew that most health care providers do not place the arm at heart level when measuring BPs. We wanted the arms resting on the bed next to the patient. The team agreed to stay together and find more conclusive answers to our research questions.

Our second study was completed in 2004 with 221 medical-surgical patients positioned supine and with the head of the bed raised 45°. Again, we noted statistically significant differences between forearm and upper arm BPs. Generally, the forearm BP was higher than the upper arm, and the differences were larger when the patient was at 45°. But we were perplexed that these differences varied from subject to subject. Not all forearm BPs were greater than upper arm BPs. Some individuals had differences less than 5mmHg while others had differences as high as 30mmHg. Indeed, forearm and upper arm BPs were not interchangeable, and because of such variation, no "magic formula" to predict upper arm pressures using forearm pressures existed. These findings confirmed hunches the team had when beginning the study. Although using forearm BPs is not best, realistically, we knew that occasions would continue to occur. Our mantra now was this: "Select the right-sized cuff, level the limb to heart level, document the site, and trend BPs using the same site!"

Soon after, we shared these findings through a second journal publication and oral and poster presentations to a wide variety of audiences, often combining the results of both studies to drive our message home. Committed to including the implications of these findings in the current hospital protocol, we were surprised that details of BP measurement and evidence to support not using forearm BPs were lacking. We quickly concluded that developing and implementing a noninvasive BP measurement clinical practice guideline (CPG) was necessary.

A subset of our team plunged into the literature on BP measurement, each member responsible for a certain aspect (e.g., body position, cuff size, manual versus oscillometric method). At this point, we were a fine-oiled machine, able to challenge and push each other to develop a quality product. After several meetings, the exchange of literature findings, consultation with experts such as physicians and IV nurses, and painstaking attention to detail of each step of taking a BP, the CPG on noninvasive BP measurement emerged! We leveled the strength of the evidence to support each section of the CPG. Photos clarified arm positioning. Following approval of the hospital's Nursing Practice Council, we began system-wide education in October 2005. This included mandatory web education, flyers, posters, and laminated cards with key points from the CPG to attach to each automatic BP monitor. To combat the challenges nurses have in finding the correct-sized cuff, particularly large cuffs, we provided nurse managers with informational packets that included suggestions and ordering information for a wide range of cuff sizes.

About that same time, our team was asked to develop the American Association of Critical-Care Nurses' (AACN) *Practice Alert: Noninvasive Blood Pressure Monitoring*. Further literature review ensued because this evidence-based document needed to be succinct and up-to-date. Sections titled "Expected Practice," "Supporting Evidence," and "What You Should Do" were developed and included. We were proud when the *Practice Alert*, representing authoritative evidence to ensure excellence in practice, was released during the AACN's National Teaching Institute in May 2006.

EBP Pearl

When external evidence from research is not available to guide best practice, it is important to comprise a team who can generate either external evidence or internal evidence through outcomes management or quality improvement projects to guide best practices.

Evidence-Based Practice in a Rural Setting

–Kenneth W. Lowrance, DNP, APRN, FNP-BC
Goodall-Witcher Healthcare Foundation, Clifton, Texas
Adjunct Faculty, Texas Christian University,
Harris College of Nursing and Health Sciences, Fort Worth, Texas

Evidence-based practice has long been a guiding principle for me throughout my 33-year career as a registered nurse. For the last 18 years, I have had the privilege of working as a family nurse practitioner in a medically underserved rural area of North Central Texas where evidence-based practice has carried even more importance and value for me.

Recently I completed a Doctor of Nursing Practice (DNP) degree. As a result, I have truly realized and appreciated how crucial the implementation of evidence-based practice is and how it has positively affected patient outcomes and motivated me to strive for excellence in every aspect of patient care delivery as an advanced practice registered nurse.

As a DNP student, my capstone project involved the development of an evidence-based diabetes management protocol for nurse practitioners in a rural health clinic setting. An extensive appraisal of the evidence revealed multiple evidence-based interventions available to implement to prevent and/or delay common complications associated with diabetes. Although various interventions have been identified by research over the years, in my particular clinical setting these specific interventions were not consistently implemented, nor were they formalized into a protocol or patient care guideline format. As a result, identifying a constellation of evidence-based interventions in this setting was truly an innovation. Despite evidence-based knowledge and well-established patient management processes of care to reduce morbidity and mortality associated with diabetes, widespread quality issues have been identified in the literature regarding the delivery of care throughout the United States. My setting was no exception to this finding.

I developed a management protocol that identified specific clinical markers to be utilized in clinical management of patients with Type 2 diabetes as well as identified goals for these markers. If markers were not at goal, the providers were expected to demonstrate evidence of intensification of therapy to help the patient attain the goal or to document a rationale as to why intensification of therapy did not occur. In addition, efforts were made to deliver diabetes care in exclusive blocks of time separate from other clinic presentations to avoid distractions and to enable the provider to focus on details of quality diabetes management.

Throughout my protocol development and through my years of experience, I have found it more and more apparent that diabetes is a labor-intensive disease, if it is to be managed appropriately. Unfortunately, many primary care providers are overwhelmed with workloads and time constraints. They do not consistently apply evidence-based principles in care. This disease is a major public health threat and is becoming epidemic. Costs of care are skyrocketing, reflecting complications resulting from poor control of the disease process and routine care of these patients. Clinical inertia, or the failure to intensify therapy when goals are not met, contributes to increased complications. The basis for protocol development was the belief that providers who apply evidence-based strategies will have improved patient outcomes and reduced or stabilized costs of care.

My rural, medically underserved practice setting serves a high percentage of Hispanic patients, many of whom are undocumented aliens and many of whom suffer from diabetes. Poverty is rampant. Implementation of the evidence-based protocol for Type 2 diabetes provided challenges because of language barriers, low socioeconomic status, and impaired health literacy. Likewise, in addition to patients with diabetes, the clinic treats a high volume of other patients, which challenges time management. Despite barriers, these challenges can be transcended by implementation of evidence-based strategies to yield effective care, such as a team approach, which is necessary for success. The evidence-based protocol implementation was accomplished by a multidisciplinary team involving nurse practitioners, physicians, staff nurses, a social worker, a registered dietician, laboratory personnel, and office personnel. All were educated regarding issues surrounding diabetes care, and all worked together to implement the translational project of evidence-based management of diabetes in a rural health clinic setting.

We provided educational interventions for the interdisciplinary participants that resulted in enhanced awareness of issues related to diabetes management. Team members felt empowered in their roles to participate in diabetes care, realizing the value of the evidence and the likely potential for improved patient outcomes. We experienced good acceptance and compliance with elements of the protocol. We assessed our outcomes on an ongoing basis, and initially those outcomes have been deemed positive.

Generally speaking, I determined that care for patients with diabetes has tremendous potential for evidence translators, implementers, and generators (i.e., researchers). Translators, as demonstrated by this project, can take research evidence and formulate protocols or patient care guidelines to assure optimal care for patients with diabetes. Evidence translators and implementers have a major impact on health care outcomes and costs. For example, adherence to components of the evidence-based management protocol would likely contribute to positive patient outcomes thereby preventing or delaying complications and decreasing associated costs. Without doubt, evidence generators, the researchers, have vast opportunities to contribute to the body of knowledge regarding care of these patients. Ongoing studies regarding new innovative interventions, their associated patient outcomes, and costs of care provide infinite opportunities for empiric study, which can benefit society at large.

We know that diabetes presents a major health threat. We know that evidence-based care truly makes a positive impact. I know that this evidence translation project, involving a protocol developed to guide care provided by nurse practitioners in a rural health clinic setting, promises to improve care for the clinic's diabetic population and can be applied in other settings.

The point, however, is that evidence-based practice is essential for quality care regardless of the setting and regardless of the disease process in question. Considerable evidence exists, and more is being produced constantly, addressing many aspects of practice. Having knowledge and skills to acquire the latest evidence is important. Having the professional drive and motivation to utilize evidence-based strategies is even more important. Not only does evidence-based practice positively affect patient outcomes, implementing it and having an awareness of its positive effect on patients is rewarding and motivating for providers. I know for me, utilizing evidence-based practices in my delivery of primary care is personally gratifying and serves to motivate me to achieve excellence in all aspects of patient care.

EBP Pearl

Use evidence, use Evidence, USE EVIDENCE, and evaluate outcome!

A Heel Pressure Ulcer Prevention Project

–Karen Boatright, MSN, RN, CNS
Clincal Nurse Specialist
VA Palo Alto Healthcare System
Menlo Park Division
Menlo Park, California

–Cherina Tinio, MSN, RN, CNS,
Clinical Coordinator
VA Palo Alto Healthcare System
Menlo Park Division
Menlo Park, California

Pressure ulcers are an unfortunate occurrence in nursing homes that can be prevented by making use of evidence-based educational programs for all nursing staff and certified nursing assistants (CNAs) who provide the bulk of physical nursing care. The heels are a common site for pressure ulcers because of the limited amount of blood flow and protective subcutaneous tissue between the skin and bone. Pressure ulcers are costly and painful, and they lengthen hospital stays. Heel ulcers are difficult to resolve and can lead to infections and surgical interventions, including amputations. The Joint Commission 2009 National Patient Safety Goals include pressure ulcer prevention as a priority for long-term care residents and requires nursing staff to take action to prevent their occurrence.

Our Heel Ulcer Prevention project was adapted from a research study conducted at the Baptist Princeton Hospital in Alabama and coordinated by a certified wound care ostomy nurse who compared the use of standard heel pillows with a heel cushion product. The project was replicated in our Community Living Center and compared standard pillows and the Sage Prevalon Heel Boot for heel offloading.

The primary goal of this heel ulcer prevention project was to implement a program that gave nursing assistants the tools needed to implement evidence-based preventative measures that could lead to a decrease in the occurrence of heel ulcers in our long-term care population. Clinical nurse specialists (CNS) performed an electronic record search to select residents who met the following selection criteria: a Braden Scale score of 6–18; intact heels; a medical diagnosis of SCI, CVA, dementia, or Parkinson's disease; and a length of stay greater than 3 months. Twenty residents were selected to participate in the 3-month project. Prior to implementation of the project, the CNS presented a 30-minute educational inservice to the nursing assistant "unit champions" via PowerPoint and a hands-on demonstration that was reinforced by the Sage Prevalon Boot vendor. Specially designated pillowcases with colorful footprints were used to designate the heel offloading pillows. The CNAs documented every shift, whether the pillows or boots were in place, and the heels were properly offloaded. The Heel Ulcer Prevention Log was placed in the activities of daily living (ADL) binder for easy access and included a comment section for additional observations. The CNS made weekly heel rounds with the CNAs to complete a skin assessment and check for proper placement of offloading devices. Two participants were discharged and one expired prior to the completion of the 3-month period. An additional two residents withdrew because of discomfort wearing the Sage Prevalon Boots and were replaced with two other residents who fit the selection criteria.

None of the participants developed heel ulcers. The CNAs became enthusiastic and empowered about their role in pressure ulcer prevention and communicated their ideas and observations to the CNS. Some of the limitations observed were incorrect application of the Sage Prevalon Boots and incomplete documentation, both of which improved as the project progressed. We found that some residents preferred the standard pillows for offloading and that no one product is for everyone. At the completion of the project, the unit champions were recognized with a certificate of appreciation presented before their peers and supervisors.

EBP Pearl

Involvement and recognition of all team members is important to successful implementation of evidence-based practice.

Best for Moms and Babies

–Vickie Wenzl, RN, AND
–Vickie Waymire, MSN, RNC, APRN-CNS
–Peggy Cline, MSN, RNC, APNR-CNS
Saint Elizabeth Regional Medical Center, Lincoln, Nebraska

Over the last several years, a phenomenon of "Birth on Demand" became firmly entrenched in Lincoln, Nebraska. It became an accepted practice to schedule the birth of a baby to accommodate busy lifestyles or to plan for relatives and friends who lived far away to participate in the happy occasion. Induction rates climbed to over 30% and inductions as early as 37 weeks were common.

Nurses came to work and were disheartened to find all the rooms full with long, slow inductions and the calendar backed up with moms waiting to come in. Providers were frustrated because they could not get their patients in at the times they desired. Team coordinators felt the brunt of the scheduling chaos, spending hours juggling physician, midwife, and patient schedules with available openings. Tenured nurses compared the labor ward of "then" and "now" and felt something was terribly amiss.

Hospital administrators, physicians, midwives, and labor and delivery nurses became increasingly uncomfortable with early inductions performed without clear medical indications. A growing body of evidence pointed to increased risk for longer labor and the need for Cesarean delivery when induction occurred early and the cervix was not ripe. In addition, the risk of premature delivery, admission to the NICU, respiratory distress syndrome, and ventilator usage increased with elective delivery prior to 39 weeks.

In January of 2007, the two medical centers delivering babies in Lincoln, Nebraska, decided to collaboratively explore the Institute for Healthcare Improvement (IHI) Idealized Design of Perinatal Care. The Idealized Design is an innovative project based on the principles of reliability science to improve care. Part of the Idealized Design is the inclusion of the Elective Induction Bundle and the Augmentation Bundle. Care bundles are a group of evidence-based interventions that when executed together result in better outcomes and a new level of safe care. Both medical center administrations and the obstetric providers recognized that if only a few decided to refuse to electively induce prior to 39 weeks, the potential existed for a family to change providers late in pregnancy to be induced on their day of choice. This would not be in the best interest of quality obstetrical care.

A core group of interested physicians, midwives, and nurses representing both medical centers came together. Each administration provided IHI membership, and the core group traveled to Boston to participate in the Impact Community presentations. Hospitals that had been a part of the Impact Community for some time shared their success stories. The enthusiasm was contagious! The Lincoln teams discussed bundle definitions and implementation strategies. The mantra that guided the Lincoln core team was "Everybody has the Same Rules." Maintaining continuity on both campuses was important to give the Lincoln community a unified message. Every pregnant woman, every office and labor and delivery nurse, and every provider would see the bundle components in the same light.

After the Boston IHI Impact Community Meeting, the challenge was to spread the enthusiasm for the possibilities that the Idealized Design offered. Change is difficult. The OB Committees at each medical center tentatively agreed to implement the Perinatal Bundles. Both facilities agreed to support a ban on elective inductions prior to 39 weeks to take the heat off the providers. They could say to an insistent pregnant woman, "The medical centers will not let me schedule you before 39 weeks."

The road to compliance was not without difficulties. For example, though they agreed with most components of the bundles, not all providers supported the 39-week limit. Some lobbied for 38.4 weeks, saying, "What difference does a few days make?" However, the core group stood firm, believing that IHI built the bundles on the strongest evidence available to guide practice.

Nurses at both medical centers quickly became strong supporters of the bundles. It was exciting to work collaboratively with a competitor for the common good of mothers and babies. Frustration born of inducing women for long hours whose bodies were not yet ready for labor changed to excitement as more and more women came into the labor and delivery unit in spontaneous labor. Nurses frequently talk to pregnant women about the benefits of waiting to 39–40 weeks: "I know you are tired of being pregnant, but the evidence shows that you and your baby will do better if you go just a little longer. I know you can do it for your baby!" Nurses quickly adopted other elements of the bundles and became increasingly skilled at titrating oxytocin in induction and augmentation of labor to avoid overstimulation of the uterus to maintain reassuring fetal status.

Fifteen months have passed since the first discussions about the IHI initiative. The changes that have occurred can be described as incredible. Over those months, the total induction rates for those moms less then 39 weeks dropped from over 30% to less than 15%. Elective inductions less than 39 weeks have been eliminated leaving only those with clear medical indications.

The rate of Cesarean delivery of induced primigravidas (i.e., first-time moms) who are greater than 39 weeks dropped from over 40% to around 20%. This is especially important because a repeat Cesarean for a woman's future pregnancies is currently the norm. A decrease in primary Cesareans is a strong strategy to reduce the overall Cesarean rate.

The nursing staff has a sense of pride and accomplishment that they participated in a large project with strong evidence guiding practice. Nurses, midwives, and physicians are experiencing a new camaraderie in working toward shared goals. Nurses have rediscovered the excitement of working with the natural forces of labor versus forcing nature.

They are reenergized by sharing in the beauty of a uniquely feminine gift—giving birth as nature intended. And they are celebrating that within a year a culture of "Birth on Demand" has changed to a culture truly based on what is "Best for Moms and Babies."

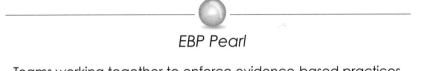

EBP Pearl

Teams working together to enforce evidence-based practices produce amazing patient outcomes.

Using Evidence-Based Practice in the Community

–*Laura Jakob, BScN, MPH*
Research Associate
Saint Elizabeth Health Care, Markham, Ontario, Canada

–*Karen Ray, RN, MSc*
Research Manager
Saint Elizabeth Health Care, Markham, Ontario, Canada

Working as a community nurse and visiting clients in their home to deliver care is a unique way of nursing. It provides the opportunity to "know" a client in a different way. Going into someone's home allows for the development of an intimate client relationship that is hard to achieve in an institutional setting. In the home, we can see pictures on the wall, smell the aromas coming from the kitchen, meet client caregivers and companions, and learn about how the client lives. As a nonprofit, home, and community care provider, Saint Elizabeth Health Care (Saint Elizabeth) has helped nurses to provide this type of care for over 100 years.

The organization has a long history of using evidence-based practice to guide its work so that clients are provided with the best care possible. It has a culture that values research and evidence and believes that it is an integral element of the nursing process. As a result, it has been recognized as Best Practice Spotlight Organization by the Registered Nurses' Association of Ontario (RNAO). This means that it has the organizational supports and infrastructures to disseminate, implement, and evaluate best practice guidelines. This is essential because working in the community means that, as nurses, we must work independently. We rely heavily on our assessment skills and judgment and must know when it's appropriate to seek clarification and guidance from others.

This independent nursing practice is one of the greatest strengths and challenges of working in home care nursing. No buildings house our supplies and technology; we have no staff room where we as nurses can gather to provide detailed information on clients at the end of a shift. Instead, home care nurses are out in the community providing care. Tracking the impact of that care in this environment can sometimes be difficult. The inability to measure and report on the outcomes of nursing in an objective way is certainly not unique to the community. All settings share a general lack of quantitative information. To address this in our setting, Saint Elizabeth decided to adopt a tool called Health Outcomes for Better Information and Care (HOBIC).

The HOBIC tool was developed by nurses for nurses and is based on evidence identified through work undertaken by an expert panel. They reviewed the literature and previous work to identify outcomes and measures that are sensitive to nursing care. These outcomes are defined by researchers and theorists as relevant to the nursing profession's scope of practice and foster a concern about what nurses do and how that impacts outcomes. Four different sections of the tool assess areas such as functional status, symptom management, patient safety, and therapeutic self-care outcomes. Each of the items on the HOBIC scale has been established as valid and reliable, is clearly defined and based on the evidence, and is linked to nursing (http://www.health.gov.on.ca/english/providers/project/hobic/measures.html).

Measurement of these specific outcomes not only helps nurses to ensure that we are undertaking a thorough assessment of client status but also allows us to have information about how clients are progressing based on our nursing care. This internal evidence is information from real clients that helps us determine if what we are doing is working or if we need to change our approach to care.

Collecting HOBIC measures and utilizing evidence in our practice is important for three reasons. First, it provides information for each nurse about how the client is progressing to meet their health care goals. It also allows administrators to use the information to identify patterns, achievements, and areas of improvement in practice. Finally, it allows the nursing profession as a whole to record and use objective, quantitative outcome measures to report on the impact of nursing and use of evidence in practice. We began using HOBIC measures in nursing in June 2009. A small team was taught how to use the tool on an electronic tablet and how to use the outcome data to inform our nursing practice. Since then, over 300 nurses have been trained to collect HOBIC outcomes and have integrated it into their nursing care. It hasn't been easy; some nurses have had reservations about using it in their practice and were unsure of the benefits it could have in improving client care. But slowly the HOBIC tool has gained support, and the tool is now utilized by more and more nurses.

What has been remarkable is how the use of HOBIC has inspired nurses to improve care. One Saint Elizabeth nurse who became very adept with the tool and incorporated it into her practice says that "just documenting and assessing these outcomes can help us really gear our care towards the patients (needs)." Another nurse who has embraced the HOBIC tool says that she has found the therapeutic self-care questions the most valuable aspect of the tool. These questions assess a client's ability to self-manage their medications, symptoms, and health planning. They provide an indication of how safe a client is in this regard. Importantly, assessing this helps identify and prevent errors that could result in serious adverse consequences for our clients. A significant amount of evidence illustrates how the period after a hospital discharge to home can be a time of great risk for medication errors. These issues may be due to error or discontinuation of medicines to monitor chronic conditions or because our client may not have a clear understanding of what drugs they are now to be taking and why. The HOBIC tool helps our team identify where there might be a concern, actively address it, and measure our clients' level of understanding, the importance of which cannot be underestimated.

One nurse said, "I can assess the client's comprehension levels and do my teaching, and then when I do the assessment again later I can assess how well they've understood the information I've given them…. It gives me a sense of accomplishment in that you know that you are leaving them in good hands and they can take care of themselves with regard to their medications."

The value of incorporating these evidence-based measures into our practice has been significant, and we are continuing to learn about how this information can help us provide better care both individually as nurses and as an organization. What is clear is that we have seen improvements in patient care as a direct result of using the HOBIC tool and that more nurses are reporting that having this evidence is translating to positive results for clients. Being able to see documented outcomes and client progression over time has provided us with a sense of accomplishment about the significance of our work, and we are excited to continue to learn about how it can help us provide better care and understand how our nursing interventions help our clients.

EBP Pearl

Evidence-based practice applies to the gamut of health care delivery.

Jacinda: An Honored Nurse Colleague

–Joya Pickett, MSN, CCNS, ACNS-BC, CCRN
System, Critical Care Clinical Nurse Specialist
Swedish Medical Center, Seattle, Washington

What follows is the account of an acute event in the life of Jacie, one of my colleagues. Jacie, a 52-year-old nurse, had just left her usual night shift in the electronic intensive care unit (eICU). Working in the eICU, often compared to being an air-traffic controller, requires constant monitoring and troubleshooting of multiple ICUs, and after all the beeps, beeps, and beeps, she was ready to drive home and get some rest. She left the hospital and went down to the second level in the parking garage where she had parked her car. Although she was feeling just fine 30 minutes before the end of her shift, she was found slumped over by the side of her car. While on their way home, family members of one of the ICU patients noted her motionless body. After determining that she was unresponsive, the visitor immediately initiated CPR and sent his wife to call for help on the emergency parking-lot phone. Both 911 emergency medical services (EMS) and the hospital Code Blue team were summoned to the scene.

As the Code Blue team arrived, CPR was still in progress; Jacie had no pulse and no spontaneous respirations. Members of the hospital code team swept in to replace the visitor who was performing CPR. The EMS team attempted intubation and because of difficulty visualizing the airway, they had to attempt a second time. Peripheral lines were started, and she immediately received epinephrine. The defibrillator pads were placed, and she was noted to be in ventricular fibrillation. Amiodarone was ordered and administered with no response. Jacie needed to be defibrillated. Less than an hour before, from the remote ICU, Jacie had just worked alongside the very nurse that was now defibrillating and shocking her back to life. She was shocked twice with 200 joules of biphasic energy. She came back in a slow but palpable pulse.

Jacie was taken directly to the ICU via a slider board, attended to by both EMS and the Code Blue team. Upon arrival to the ICU she had no spontaneous movement, was unresponsive to deep pain, and had decerebrate posturing to stimuli. Her pupils were equal and reactive to light, 3+ brisk, and consensual. She was in sinus rhythm with occasional premature ventricular contractions (PVCs) with an incomplete right bundle branch block. Her heart sounds were normal except for a soft ejection murmur. The fourth-year resident attempted placment of a central line and noted an intravenous chemotherapy treatment port in the right anterior chest wall; therefore, he placed a triple lumen central line on her left side. Her lungs were clear, and a chest X-ray for endotracheal tube placement was ordered STAT. Jacie had a bump to her left temporal area and a cut just above her lip to the left. A CT scan was ordered to rule out possible head injury subsequent to her cardiac arrest and loss of consciousness, which caused her fall.

Upon admission to the ICU, one of the first questions the charge nurse asked was if Jacie was a candidate to initiate the new hypothermia cooling after ventricular fibrillation/pulseless tachycardia cardiac arrest protocol. The foundation of this evidence-based intervention is that anoxic brain injury after cardiac arrest is a major source of mortality and morbidity. A large body of evidence suggests that mild therapeutic hypothermia protects the brain during global ischemia that occurs during cardiac arrest and leads to improved neurologic outcomes. This protocol consists of placing the patient on a cooling system that carefully regulates the temperature to 33° C for a period of 24 hours. The nursing staff, having never had an indication to initiate this protocol with the new cooling device, were now advocating its use.

To consider use of this protocol, those making the decision need a thorough history and physical to consider potential inclusion and exclusion criteria. In March, just 9 months prior, Jacie went to her doctor for a routine mammogram. The right breast showed density in the upper aspect and a possible nodule in her mid-breast area. A follow-up ultrasound exam showed a suspicious lesion in the 12 o'clock region of the right breast. Ultrasound-guided core biopsy was then performed showing an infiltrating ductal carcinoma. Jacie began treatment for breast cancer with chemotherapy followed by Taxol for 12 weeks. Radiation therapy began just one week ago. Jacie's family medical history consisted of her father dying of a heart attack at age 53 and her mother who died from breast cancer.

After a careful review of Jacie's biosystems, labs, and tests, therapeutic hypothermia was ordered and promptly initiated. One of the concerns with the use of hypothermia is the masking of infection, and as Jacie has been on Neupogen, she has a history of being leukopenic. As this is a relative exclusion criterion, the plan was to move forward with therapeutic hypothermia and to vigilantly watch for signs of infection. The goal is to start therapy as soon as possible after the return of spontaneous circulation. Previously ice bags and regular cooling blankets were used; however, these devices are not as reliable at obtaining 33° C within a one-hour period. The new device is more reliable in obtaining the desired temperature rapidly and in helping to prevent overshooting to a lower temperature. Jacie's nurses measured her to identify the correct size of therapy pads. Chest and leg pads were applied and the monitor set to cool to 33° C for a 24-hour period. Jacie was placed on the cooling protocol and received pain and sedative medications for general comfort and to tolerate the cooling therapy.

Early the next morning Jacie's husband and two children, ages 16 and 17, came to see her. It was difficult to console them because their wife and mother was unresponsive with mostly reflexive motion. The multidisciplinary team talked about how Jacie had gone through a dramatic event and her body was in shock. We discussed her plan of care for the next few hours and days. As the head CT was negative for bleeding, heparin would be started, nitroglycerine would be used empirically if her blood pressure would allow, and we would continue to correct any electrolyte imbalances. We reinforced that her heart and other biosystems were stable, that she was tolerating the hypothermia therapy well, and that all signs indicated that she was headed in the right direction. The major goals were to assess and hope for signs of neurologic recovery over the next few days.

Jacie quickly showed dramatic improvement. Controlled rewarming occurred the next day over a 6–8 hour period, and although she was still unresponsive, she remained stable. As her sedative medications were weaned down, she began to have spontaneous and purposeful movements. She was extubated without event on day three. Though slow at first, she soon began to respond to commands. By the evening of day 4, Jacie stated, "I'm feeling much better, but I continue to feel 'foggy.'"

Results from Jacie's tests were all coming together. She had a minimal rise in her cardiac enzymes considered related to the arrest, her angiogram was negative, and an echocardiogram demonstrated normal overall left ventricular function. Therefore, it was determined that the cause of Jacie's cardiac arrest was a primary ventricular fibrillation arrhythmia. Insertion of an automatic internal cardio defibrillator (AICD) was recommended. After discussion with her oncologist, those in charge of her care decided it would have to be placed on her left side because she was receiving both chemotherapy and radiation therapy to her right side. The hope was that on the left side it would be shielded enough that the device would not be in conflict with her radiation therapy. Confounding this decision was the knowledge that she would not be able to receive MRIs in the future for follow-up analysis of her cancer treatments. On day 10, Jacie had her AICD placed.

Jacie is now back at work and sharing her enthusiasm for life with her patients. She is working in the outpatient chemotherapy treatment unit. Jacie is tireless in the care she provides her patients. She feels that her own experience with cancer and her recent experience in the ICU can help her patients to feel hope and inspiration. She is a good listener, and by listening, she teaches her patients that their thoughts and opinions matter. In everything that she does, she teaches us to treat others with respect and dignity. Her actions embody the profession of nursing, as she is a compassionate person with a keen sense of providing safe evidence-based care to her patients.

The multidisciplinary team identified three things that were beneficial in promoting improved outcomes for Jacie: (1) the visitor's prompt initiation of CPR; (2) early defibrillation; and (3) the early initiation of hypothermia—all evidence-based interventions with reliable outcomes. Though therapeutic hypothermia is likely to have directly contributed to Jacie's neurological outcomes, the support of her family and the staff and her own passion for living were paramount to her full recovery.

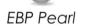

EBP Pearl

Evidence-based solutions bring excellent outcomes!

Real-Life EBP: A Front-line Staff Affair

–Shirley A. Storch Sherman, MN, RN, CCRN
Critical Care Assistant Nurse Manager
Virginia Mason Medical Center, Seattle, Washington

I first heard about "evidence-based practice" at a nurse research conference in Seattle from Dr. Marita Titler, the keynote speaker. She spoke about the Iowa Model and the process to engage front-line staff. It was totally logical to me to involve staff for innovation, implementation, and acceptance of a practice change. It also provided rationale through clinical inquiry and discovery by the staff nurse. The Iowa Model and the concept of evidence-based practice took me on my own personal exploration for professional growth and staff development.

As I started my own quest to learn more about evidence-based practice (EBP), Melnyk and Fineout-Overholt's publications appeared frequently in my literature searches. I also found Titler's work on EBP referenced throughout the literature. I embarked on a graduate degree in nursing and incorporated the application of EBP in my studies and in my organization for quality improvement because the topic aligned so well with both entities.

Anna Gawlinski, RN, Director of Evidence-Based Practice at UCLA Medical Center, also has provided a structure for front-line staff involvement in EBP and research. Her development of a model to have staff participation without leaving the bedside has demonstrated the importance of including a very influential and vital group from the initiation of an idea to completion of a quality improvement or research project.

With such exemplar role models on EBP and my deliberate attempt to involve staff nurses, I was off to a reassuring start with my own EBP endeavors for school and work. That work focuses on the significant nursing management problem of delirium in the critical-care patient. Delirium has been accepted as an unfortunate, but unavoidable risk. Delirium has been labeled "ICU psychosis" or "ICU syndrome," and in the critically ill it can occur in up to 87% of mechanically ventilated patients.

Acute illness coupled with sedation, immobility, and the hospital environment has been correlated with the increased incidence of delirium. Delirium runs the gamut of cognitive impairment, which includes an altered level of consciousness, disorganized thinking, inattention, and a fluctuating mental status from a patient's baseline. Delirium has been associated with reintubation, increased length of stay and costs, morbidity, and lasting cognitive impairment. Modifiable risk factors have been identified to reduce the prevalence of delirium and provide direction for prevention and treatment. The data were too compelling to ignore.

Delirium monitoring in critical care has been a relentless drumbeat for Dr. Wes Ely and Brenda Pun, RN, and their research colleagues at Vanderbilt. The research on the impact of delirium in critical care clearly validated the need to implement delirium monitoring and not omit the staff to get the project accepted and completed. Reading the assigned and nonassigned publications of the EBP gurus Drs. Melnyk, Fineout-Overholt, and Titler, and quality improvement czar Dr. Donald Berwick, I methodically planned a timeline that not only included staff nurses, but also a collaborative team of physician and pharmacy champions. Barriers to acceptance of translational research and implementation of the evidence-based variations in one's own practice can be related to not understanding the value and reasoning of change in practice.

The opportunity to go to the EBP or research "mecca" before commencing on a practice change to experience the passion and visualize the operations is priceless. So, off we went to Nashville to partake in some country music, southern cooking, and delirium monitoring in critical care. Along with meeting the research experts of delirium, the travel team of bedside nurses, a physician champion, and I were able to tour the critical-care unit and talk to the nurses on how they documented and incorporated the assessment to reduce the risk of delirium development when caring for their patients. Besides receiving our own personal presentation by Dr. Ely, we were told we would receive assistance in implementing the evidence-based protocol of delirium monitoring in our critical-care unit.

The energy that was emitted from the travel team was contagious and evoked curiosity from the home team. What was "CAM-ICU"? Why was delirium so dangerous? What could a bedside nurse do to prevent something that was accepted as "part of doing business," such as pressure ulcers, bloodstream infections, and ventilator-associated pneumonia were before evidence-based practices were implemented? I became the facilitator of the project instead of the terminator of change because of my leadership position in the unit. Providing the evidence, rationale, support, and resources along with mentoring and coaching front-line staff involved with quality improvement work were my mission and role.

Two studies provided guidance for implementation of an evidence-based protocol for delirium at the bedside. Devlin and colleagues proposed that a combined education intervention consisting of didactic learning and scenarios assists with delirium assessment skills of the bedside practitioner. Pun implemented delirium and sedation monitoring in two medical centers' critical care units. Inservices with case studies, handouts, pocket cards, and discussion at bedside rounds and modification in electronic documentation for compliance provided a successful planned implementation process. In my quality improvement role, I provided encouragement and tidbits of advice to the "implementers" of EBP delirium monitoring.

Much to my amazement, the staff not only accepted the idea of doing another task, but also wanted electronic support to remind them to monitor for delirium reliably. The physician and pharmacy champions continued to provide up-to-date research publications to support the cause and reinforce the importance of the patient's delirium status in multidisciplinary rounds daily. The nurses were not practicing in solo. They were contributing members of the team, keeping the patient safe, improving outcomes using the most current evidence, and talking the same language as their interdisciplinary colleagues.

As my delirious EBP band of nurses were checking daily if the CAM-ICU (validated screening tool) was being used for delirium identification, the physicians and pharmacists were trialing alternative medications to reduce the risk of delirium development. As part of my scholarly project for school, I conducted a descriptive survey of nurses' perceptions post-implementation of an education intervention on delirium monitoring. A quantitative questionnaire was distributed to the nurses in my critical-care unit through SurveyMonkey. The study surveyed current practices of critical-care nurses with protocols and guidelines in place caring for patients with delirium and the significance delirium has on patient outcomes. Measuring the comprehension and beliefs of nurses who have had a practice change can be very revealing. Although "stories sell, data tells."

The critical-care nurses reported that the inability to complete a delirium assessment in a sedated patient was the most significant barrier. They agreed that delirium is underdiagnosed, a common response to the CCU environment, requires active interventions on the part of the caregivers, and is associated with higher patient mortality. My replication study findings were consistent with the Devlin study. Our next step is dissemination of the delirium-monitoring protocol throughout the hospital with the support of our administrators and front-line staff.

Berwick reports that a component of the adoption of an EBP is the dissemination of innovations that include the perception of the innovation, the characteristics of the adopters of the change, and the managerial factors of the organization. With conceptual theory as a backbone, weaving the contributions of the entire multidisciplinary team from conception to completion has guaranteed a successful endeavor for my critical-care unit and for me professionally. I am indebted to the steadfast devotion of the EBP forefathers who have provided the guidance for us to deliver the best care for the best outcomes.

EBP Pearl

Involvement of multidisciplinary team members can accelerate the implementation of evidence-based practices.

Do Research to Implement EBP and Make Your Heart Soar

–Louise Trygstad, DNSc, RN, CNS

–Robin Buccheri, DNSc, RN, MHNP

–Glenna A. Dowling, PhD, RN, FAAN
School of Nursing, University of California, San Francisco, California

–Martha D. Buffum, DNSc, RN, PMHCNS-BC
Veterans Affairs Medical Center, San Francisco, California
School of Nursing, University of California, San Francisco, California

–April A. Gerlock, PhD, RN, ARNP, PMHNP-BC, PMHCNS-BC
VA Puget Sound Health Care System, American Lake Division, Seattle and Tacoma, Washington
University of Washington, School of Nursing, Seattle, Washington

–Patricia Birmingham, RN, MS
Veterans Affairs Medical Center, San Francisco, California
School of Nursing, University of California, San Francisco, California

Our professional spirit has taken flight in the process of moving from the opportunity to have a little academic release time for research to disseminating our evidence-based practice (EBP) nationally across the Department of Veterans Affairs as a best practice! While in doctoral studies, we learned about research and research methods and completed a supervised dissertation. In working for a university where the course load was teaching 12 units each semester, we had no time to practice the research skills we had learned. Then, we were given a gift from the university: 3 units of release time each semester for research as long as we were productive!

Robin and I (LT) were students together in the doctoral program at the University of California, San Francisco (UCSF) and were both hired by the University of San Francisco the same year upon completion of our doctorates. Because we were both psychiatric nurses, it was only natural for us to explore the opportunity to conduct research together. We began searching for topics that had the potential to help patients, were in the domain of nursing, and could sustain our interest for years. After reading everything we could find in the English language about auditory hallucinations and management techniques that had been found to help persons who heard them (about an inch of articles), we chose to test nursing interventions for persistent auditory hallucinations. Robin spent a sabbatical year working with Drs. Linda Chafetz, RN (expert on schizophrenia), and Pat Larson, RN, of the Symptom Management Group—both at UCSF. Building on the extant literature, symptom management framework, adult learning theory, and research that found psychotic symptoms could be managed by patients, we developed a course: Behavioral Management of Persistent Auditory Hallucinations.

We knew we had to have tools and measurements to assess the outcomes of the course on patients, so we sought the help of Dr. Glenna Dowling, RN, an expert statistician and researcher at UCSF. We completed a pilot study of the course through collaborations with the San Francisco VA Medical Center (SFVA). We sought help from Bernice Waldron, RN, Director of the Day Treatment Center, and Dr. Nick Kanas, MD, recognized for his group work with people with schizophrenia. These three professionals made many suggestions for improving our course and research. This wonderful collaboration resulted in publications of our findings from the pilot and one year follow-up study.

When we began teaching the course to patients, we were acutely aware that we knew nothing of the experience of auditory hallucinations except what we had read. We could not answer questions from our own experience. So we told our first group that we had read everything we could about what helped for voices, and we wanted to teach them what we thought were the best ideas from what we read. We hoped that we would all teach each other—they would teach us about their experiences and what helped and what did not. We shared our own experience with symptom management. For example, I (LT) have asthma, Robin has migraines, and they hear voices; we could all learn to manage our symptoms better if we learned more about them and tried different techniques that others had found successful. This perspective of interactive learning and empowerment remains the guiding principle of our course and contributes enormously to our inspiration.

Our pilot study needed to be expanded to a larger study so we again sought consultation for design from Dr. Glenna Dowling; we planned to teach many of the classes on our sabbatical, which we did. What was clear was that we needed more classes to be taught. So we started inviting psychiatric nurses who expressed interest in our work to participate in the research with us and teach a class. This study, also with significant findings, was reported in an article with all 12 of us sharing the authorship. The 12 of us had accomplished the work together, and we learned wonderful things from our colleagues. After the follow-up study was published (again with all 12 sharing authorship), we won a Best Practice Award—Best Treatment of Schizophrenia in a Behavioral Health Care Program from the American Psychiatric Nurses Association (APNA).

It was evident now that Robin and I (LT) and a few others could teach the course with positive results. However, for the course to reach a broader patient population, we needed to demonstrate that any interested psychiatric nurse could successfully teach it. So we began working with Dr. Marti Buffum, RN (SFVA), and Dr. April Gerlock (VA Puget Sound Health Care System, Seattle and Tacoma, Washington) to plan and implement a program disseminating the course to advanced practice nurses within the VA system. We also developed a safety protocol during this process based on our findings and the need to deliberately assess whether or not patients experienced commands to harm themselves or others and whether they intended to act on those commands. We published both articles. Dissemination of our evidence is the last step in the EBP process. If we do not disseminate, others do not learn best practices to benefit their patients. Yes, nurses who receive materials and mentoring via regularly scheduled teleconferences can successfully teach the course.

Our biggest surprise and continued inspiration was how much each nurse teaching the course gave us regarding ideas/suggestions to improve the course. For example, one nurse developed a charting template and started a "graduate group." Two other nurses working together developed user-friendly homework that was used during class sessions in an interactive manner, which encourages more active patient participation. We presented poster sessions about this project, one of which was at a National Alliance on Mental Illness (NAMI) conference where the Chief for VA Mental Health Services asked us if we would disseminate this program throughout the VA. We are thrilled to be working on widespread dissemination now. After all, of what use is an effective course if no one teaches it? We also are writing a paper on the theory of persistent auditory hallucinations. Of what value is all that we have learned if we cannot pass it on? Although we all use theory and Robin teaches it, we decided to invite Trish Birmingham (UCSF doctoral candidate) to work with us and bring her fresh ideas on diagramming theory to our team.

We can measure our success in many ways: The course has been taught in many psychiatric settings throughout California, the United States, and multiple countries; we have published eight articles in peer reviewed journals and presented at many conferences, most recently at the First World Hearing Voices Congress and APNA, and give other poster sessions and many presentations at the national, state, and local level of NAMI. In November of 2010, Robin, our team leader, was inducted into the American Academy of Nursing primarily as a result of this work. Perhaps most inspirationally, at the end of the course when participants are asked about their experience, over 90% always say the course was helpful to them. Many of them have never talked openly about their voices, and they appreciate having a safe place to share their experience and hear the experience of others.

However, I (LT) would say that the real success has been in the joy of working together, with colleagues and patients, to find a way to successfully intervene to decrease the impact of a symptom that is commonly encountered by psychiatric nurses. By the way, I (LT) retired as a professor 10 years ago. As a volunteer, I am still a very active member of our team because it warms my heart and makes my spirit soar.

Lastly, if we could make suggestions to new researchers, we would say to find at least one research partner or mentor. Doing research alone seems almost impossible in both academic and clinical settings. Too many other things become priorities. Working with a research partner(s) multiplies the ideas and resources and makes research and its dissemination as EBP feasible. Collaborate with other researchers and clinicians from other disciplines and agencies (which leads to wider dissemination and earlier changes in practice) and be inclusive regarding sharing credit and resources. We have always given away what we developed (e.g., treatment manual and instruments), and we have gotten so much in return. Our hearts are soaring. If you would like to teach this course or expand this research, please contact us.

EBP Pearl

Working with partners and in teams in collaboration with patients across institutions can leverage and magnify the impact of research and evidence-based practice.

6

Mentoring and Teaching Evidence-Based Practice

Mentors are the sustaining factor for an evidence-based practice (EBP) culture. EBP mentoring is an intentional, focused effort to foster growth and excellence in care providers who make a difference in health care outcomes. Whether clinicians are learning from preceptors, colleagues, or faculty, mentorship must be the hallmark of health care education and clinical practice. This chapter shares stories about growing the best and brightest clinicians by nurturing mentors, as these clinicians are the future of health care. We all will engage the health care system at some point in our lives and will appreciate receiving the best care possible by caring clinicians who have been taught and mentored to be their absolute best at improving our health outcomes.

Mentoring is *more an affair of the heart* than the head—it is a *2-way relationship* that is based on *trust. –Tobin*

Turning Caterpillars Into Butterflies Through Evidence-Based Practice

–Carol Ann Esche, DNP, MA, RN, NE-BC
Clinical Nurse Specialist in Evidence-based Practice and Research
Franklin Square Hospital Center, Baltimore, Maryland

"You want me to do what?" nurses ask at the beginning of their evidence-based practice (EBP) internship program. Weeks later these same nurses comment, "My professional life will never be the same again." What made such a dramatic impact in the professional career of these nurses? It was learning about and incorporating EBP, including research, into their professional practice. In my role as Clinical Nurse Specialist in Evidence-based Practice and Research at Franklin Square Hospital Center, in Baltimore, Maryland, I have the privilege of mentoring nurses to improve their effectiveness in delivering patient care through the implementation of EBP. Unleashing these expert clinical nurses, yet novices to the scientific and EBP processes, is like watching caterpillars turn into beautiful butterflies spreading their wings in full glory.

One nurse, one observation, plus a little passion—that is the recipe for EBP success. Over the years, nurses have hesitantly approached me with their clinical questions, usually prefacing their observation with, "I am not sure this is important but . . ." In all my experience, I have never had one clinical question that was not important or worthy of review. Questions have ranged from the size of catheters for blood transfusions, identified by Pam, a vascular access nurse with 30 years of experience; to evaluating evidence about standardizing the back OR table, identified by Beth, a nurse in the OR; to evaluating the use of gastrostomy tube dressings by Amanda, a medical-surgical nurse. All of their questions serve as powerful testimony to the bedside staff nurses who have honed their critical-thinking skills.

Evidence-based practice is a grass-roots approach to introducing and managing change. The ability to gather data and disseminate results in the hospital, across a hospital network, and through professional organizations has accelerated the speed of change within nursing. The nursing profession is moving in tandem with other health care professions to incorporate best practices into patient care. Like planting a butterfly garden, embedding EBP into the institutional culture yields exponential results as nurses pollinate their organization with fresh ideas and new approaches to patient care.

There are three reasons why I believe that EBP has the opportunity to transform the nursing profession like never before. First, though nurses have always been diligent in care of their patients, now nurses can impact more than one or two patients at a time through EBP. For example, Gale, an RN in community health, developed an evidence-based toolkit for pediatric asthma patients to be used in our pediatric emergency department (Peds ED) and all pediatric outpatient and pediatric private practices in our hospital. Building the collaborative relationships necessary to produce this tool kit has the potential to facilitate improvement in asthmatic pediatric patient outcomes across all these settings.

Secondly, EBP, including research, provides nurses with the necessary information to confidently discuss health care issues and policies with the media, politicians, physicians, consumers, and other nurses, because nurses know that they have the best evidence at their fingertips. For example, George is working collaboratively with physicians in the ED as he determines what the evidence says about how best to manage patients with multiple comorbidities in the psychiatric ED. Other examples include Diane, a post-anesthesia care unit (PACU) nurse, who established a relationship with nurses in Australia who were also evaluating the use of mean arterial pressure in the critical care and post-anesthesia setting, and Kelly, an ICU nurse, who spoke to a crowd of over 200 people for her first professional podium presentation on caring in the ICU setting. EBP has fostered the metamorphosis of these bedside staff nurses into health care transformers who are setting higher standards in patient care.

Finally, it has been my experience that with mentorship, every nurse can become a nurse scholar. I have had nurses tell me that they want to do a rigorous EBP internship and not have a "pansy experience." When EBP projects develop into research studies, bedside staff nurses have learned how to collect data and lead the research study. For example, Li, a telemetry nurse, is leading an experimental study evaluating face-to-face and computerized education for teaching how to stage pressure ulcers. Sometimes EBP internship projects turn into educational rollouts, like it did for Ginny, who educated her peers in the ICU about the best delirium assessment tool that was supported by the evidence. As their projects have unfolded, bedside staff nurses have honed their writing skills through preparing manuscripts, developing slide presentations, and designing scientific posters to disseminate the results of their EBP projects and research studies. The smile and glow of pride when it was announced at our EBP and Research Council that Carol, a 30-year vascular access nurse, had a project accepted to present at National Database of Nursing Quality Indicators (NDNQI) will never be forgotten!

Evidence-based practice is about allowing evidence to change your practice. It is appropriate that nurses initiate EBP projects with the expectation of project outcomes. However, sometimes the results are contrary to what they expect. For example, Beth, a nurse educator at our hospital, took on the seemingly easy task of examining the use of skills fairs to evaluate staff competencies. The evidence led her in a direction that she had not expected. Beth realized that internal evidence (practice data), such as time schedules, did not support the use of skill fairs to evaluate some competencies, which corroborated the lack of external evidence (research) supporting the use of skill fairs. Given that some evidence supported the use of journaling as a competency tool, Beth evaluated it to see if it was an effective method of assessing specific competencies. Based on her results, she has introduced journaling as an option for some clinical competencies with great success on her unit.

So how do you measure EBP outcomes? One EBP project at a time! A review of our scholarly log for the past 24 months yielded approximately 9 Institutional Review Board submissions, 2 book chapters, 14 journal articles, 1 online publication, 44 EBP projects, and 100 oral or poster presentations conducted by nurses at our community hospital. You know EBP has been embedded in your organization when a director runs into your office to ask you to mentor a nurse about copyright issues. You know EBP is a success when after holding your annual EBP and Research Conference sponsored by your EBP and Research Council, a nurse decides to earn her PhD degree! Another way to measure success is when the shared governance councils want to participate in EBP, including research, to solve the issues that confront them.

A group of butterflies is called a kaleidoscope. The bright and iridescent colors of the butterfly reflect light and the changing patterns in the world about them. Bedside nurses, too, are like a kaleidoscope as we reflect the light of new internal and external evidence in our daily practice. My charge to all of us is for the nursing profession to continue to meet the challenges of complex patient care through the careful integration of EBP into our daily decision-making.

EBP Pearl

Organizational cultures will shift with persistent, mentored EBP!

Teaching EBP: Bridging Practice and Scholarship

–Kathleen Neville, PhD, RN
Professor, School of Nursing
Kean University, Union, New Jersey

Evidence-based practice (EBP) has not just inspired the RN-BSN students that I teach, it has also greatly inspired me, and I believe it has made me a far more effective educator. Rather than use the term *inspiration* for my perception of how EBP has influenced RN-BSN nurses and their education at my institution, I think a more fitting statement might be that EBP has created a "reinfusion of enthusiasm towards practice" for RN-BSN students. As I reflect on this creative journey in exploring EBP and becoming a champion of EBP in my academic setting, it's hard to believe that it has been nearly 6 years since I first learned about EBP and hard to imagine how with each year it is becoming more firmly integrated into our undergraduate program.

My initial exposure to EBP was really memorable because I immediately became absolutely enthralled with EBP! So the story begins. In 2004, my chairperson at Kean University School of Nursing asked if I could attend an American Association of Colleges of Nursing conference in Miami. It was undoubtedly an eye-opening experience for me as two monumental changes in nursing were addressed at the meeting: first, the introduction of the DNP as a terminal clinical degree in nursing and, second, the keynote presentation of evidence-based practice by Bernadette Melnyk. Having been educated to be a researcher and having also been a long-time course leader of the research courses at my institution, I was well aware of the difficulties, challenges, and obstacles for nurses in the conduct of research and, more importantly, of the real disconnect students perceived when I spoke about the dramatic advances in nursing research and theory development. Despite my passion for research and my focus on presenting nursing's progress in the conduct of rigorous nursing research over the past 30 years and the importance of research for furthering nursing science, many nurses in our program described research as removed from their practice and indicated that their conduct of or involvement with research in daily practice was practically nonexistent. So when I heard this initial presentation of EBP and how it so seamlessly provided the mechanism for nurses to accessibly use research evidence in their practice, I knew it was the answer to my concerns about teaching research to undergraduate students. One lecture and I was on a mission to gain more knowledge about EBP.

It was during that conference in that presentation that I realized that EBP was exactly what was needed in nursing to advance scholarly practice so that nurses in clinical practice could easily retrieve the best evidence and use it in a timely manner to plan the best care. EBP was the vehicle to bridge scholarship and practice. Two months later, at the inception of the spring semester, I introduced the idea of conducting a pilot study to a group of creative, intellectually curious students to explore the implementation of EBP in our RN-BSN program. Students were just as excited as I was. It was an ideal environment for learning because the ambiance was one of creative, stimulating collegiality as I communicated early on in the course that I too was a learner and that we would all be involved in collaborative learning along with one of our reference librarians who was also most enthusiastic and intrigued to learn about EBP.

Nurses immediately became engaged in learning about EBP; steadfastly drafted, formulated, and revised PICO questions; and in collaboration with our reference librarian began retrieval of the best evidence for questions regarding their current clinical practice. Evidence appraisal and synthesis of the literature with clinical decision-making in consideration of the level of evidence, patient preferences and values, and health care expertise then followed.

Topics and subsequent PICO questions were diverse and reflected questions posed from their clinical practice. For example, pediatric telephone triage nurses who identified a lack of standard protocol for parental instructions on antipyretic use in school-age children with fever explored the best evidence regarding selection of OTC medication. Nurses employed on a medical-surgical unit posed the following PICO question: In elderly hospitalized patients, how do physical restraints compared to bed monitor/sensors affect falls prevention? Oncology nurses interested in the psychosocial aspects of illness explored the evidence that demonstrated the efficacy of follow-up telephone support services after outpatient visits and formulated the following PICO question: In patients undergoing outpatient chemotherapy, how does follow-up telephone support and psychosocial education compared to the standard nursing intervention affect anxiety during outpatient services?

Other PICO questions addressed comparing nursing interventions such as (a) how dressing types affected central venous catheter infections and management of skin tears in elderly clients in long-term care facilities; (b) how prophylaxis interventions affected incidence of deep vein thrombosis in surgical patients; and (c) how parental educational nursing interventions affected urinary tract infections in uncircumcised preschool male children.

Through this learning opportunity of implementing EBP into our curriculum, I found several issues became more evident. A key component in the RN-BSN curriculum is the inclusion of content to foster knowledge and skills for nurses to become designers and managers of nursing care, which necessitates that nurses use critical thinking in decision-making. In my own personal experience as an RN-BSN student transitioning into a BSN program, I had previously been taught to defer many decisions to others. As an educator, I have witnessed this hesitancy and reticence in decision-making among RN-BSN students in previous years. However, upon implementation of EBP in our curriculum, and with students immersed in critical appraisal and synthesis of the literature, I noticed that their ability to confidently make clinical decisions soared and soon became the norm. Quite a feat!

Another advantage of using EBP in our curriculum was that through the close collaboration with the students engaging in EBP projects, I became more closely aware of their learning needs, and it became easier to identify students in need of further support, whether it pertained to their ability to perform efficient searches, to recognize the best literature, or to critically appraise the literature and determine the best practice. Students faced challenges in that unfamiliar topics or interventions required substantial reading before they could determine the most relevant PICO question (i.e., background information). However, the benefit was that nurses clearly experienced the professional role of nursing as they identified the state of the scientific knowledge as the best way of knowing rather than relying on tradition, authority, or trial and error to guide their practice decisions. Witnessing nurses becoming more confident and assertive and displaying stronger professional behaviors through their EBP projects was extremely gratifying and rewarding.

RN-BSN student responses to EBP were equally positive. Students clearly identified the value of using EBP in practice, and many students brought their knowledge gained about EBP to their institutions and embarked on the role of EBP champion. Here are some of the students' views about their experience of learning EBP in our program:

> *"I actually had fun researching, collaborating with my partner and faculty, and discovering evidence regarding our project. I learned the importance of nurses knowing how to use current research in their practice. I would like to continue EBP projects to increase my knowledge, improve patient outcomes, and influence the profession of nursing."*

> *"Learning EBP has made me realize how important it is to my daily practice and how much more needs to be done."*

> *"I am now better prepared to use research in my practice, and I am excited to inform my coworkers what I have learned and relay the importance of reading research evidence and applying it to our practice."*

> *"This EBP project has helped me realize the importance of research and of using evidence to educate other health care staff, patients, and families as well. Learning how to access the best evidence available to appropriately implement care has all been part of this course which has encouraged me to better evaluate articles and be able to give my patients more expertise in their care."*

> *"I now have more awareness of research and EBP and feel I have more confidence to join committees in my hospital."*

> *"This project reinforced the need for RNs to be involved in evidence-based practice to determine the best standards of care and professional practice."*

EBP has now become standard in our curriculum, and the increased interest and involvement among faculty, students, and the agencies that benefit from these EBP projects continues to grow with each year that we become more experienced in this new paradigm. New discoveries and challenges will undoubtedly occur in our evolving pursuit of teaching EBP, but the creative, intellectually stimulating milieu generated by bridging practice and scholarship through EBP has not only provided improved patient outcomes, but also has reinfused much enthusiasm and positive energy in my teaching. With anticipation, I look forward to increased student-faculty involvement with creative EBP projects.

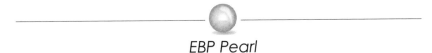

EBP Pearl

Nursing students want to learn about EBP, and they want to implement the process and paradigm in practice!

Research and EBP: Not as Easy as 1-2-3, but Worth It to Make a Difference

–Carol Victor, RN-C, CDE
Advocate Lutheran General Hospital
Park Ridge, Illinois

Our journey into evidence-based practice (EBP) started one day at a professional development meeting when the group was asked, "Who would be interested in delving into nursing research?" After a few minutes of downcast eyes and silence, four timid hands went up. Little did we know that these pioneer women would still be together 4 years later, continuing to work at learning how to conduct research and implement EBP.

Our initial project was to replicate a study about nurse identification originally conducted at Rush-Copley Medical Center. For our team, the study actually took a backseat to the process. We wanted to learn how to do EBP and the process of nursing research. After all, we did volunteer.

Our team consisted of three dedicated advanced practice nurses (APNs) whose charge was to mentor the four bedside nurses into the realm of nursing research. Our group was diverse, consisting of representation from pediatrics, medical nursing, cardiovascular diagnostics, and obstetrics. This diversity added to our ability to bring different perspectives to the table. We were novices, and without the theoretical handholding by these intelligent and unbelievably patient APNs, we would not have gotten off the ground.

Our first of many stumbling blocks was the time expectation. We were given one year to complete our study. Our team was in the spotlight because this research project was the first one to be funded by the Nursing Endowment Committee at Advocate Lutheran General Hospital (ALGH), our hospital. One of the most valuable lessons we learned was that research takes an incredible amount of time. Because our study consisted of direct patient and family interviews about their preferences for nurse identification, finding appropriate patients and families was at many times difficult.

Attempting to get patients and families to agree to yet one more questionnaire was an obstacle we faced boldly. In retrospect, this was a daunting task, because we were recruiting and surveying patients after our workday was complete, and many times we wished for an incentive to help with participation. Finally the day came when we had surveyed all of our targeted 240 patients.

With our patient surveys complete, it was time to tabulate the results. Statistics? No one said that math would be involved in this! Now what would we do? Could we make sense out of this data or was our work in vain? Behold, our mentors showed us the yellow brick road to reality and introduced us to a statistician. We were fortunate enough to have a statistician at our institution who provided us with excellent insight.

After tabulation of the results, lo and behold, our study results demonstrated that the patients and families surveyed preferred a "red and white nursing badge" as a means of identifying their nurse. We shared the results of this study with nursing administration who endorsed the incorporation of the "nurse badge" for all registered nurses at ALGH and Advocate Lutheran General Children's Hospital (ALGCH). The "nurse badges" were distributed during Nurses Week in May 2008.

Now, we truly thought we were done and could finally take a respite. However, the story was really just unfolding. Little did we know the impact that the nurse badge would have on our institution. The president of the medical staff was so impressed with the easy identification of a nurse demonstrated by the red and white nursing badge that he wanted this for the physicians as well. The wearing of colored badges is now common practice in our institution, and to our delight, all disciplines are now sporting badges of many colors. This practice has added to the ease of identification of all health care personnel at our institution, thus improving patient and staff satisfaction. Clearly identifying all health care providers interacting with patients and families is important, and the colored badges worn daily at our institution are a continual reminder that nursing research and EBP do "make a difference."

Our group has continued to evolve. We have been fortunate that this diverse group of nurses "jelled" and are committed to working together. The process of mentoring is continuing, and our next nursing study will involve the bedside nurses taking the lead on an evidence-based project with the APNs as true mentors. Like any parent or seasoned nurse knows, allowing mistakes to happen all for the sake of learning is often difficult and sometimes painful. In the true spirit of mentorship, our APN mentors have allowed us to stumble and fall. However, they are always there to pick us up, dust us off, and get us back on the right path. One of our take-home messages from all this stumbling and falling is that participation in a replication study does not a nursing researcher make. As a novice in the EBP process, you need experience and guidance on your side. You need a mentor. However, despite all of our missteps and misfires, our spirit is strong. We are not giving up.

After completion of the nurse badge study, our team worked together to develop a "perfect manuscript" and to chose the right journal for submission. Imagine our dismay when we were rejected. So we regrouped, rewrote, and submitted to another journal. Alas, rejection again.

Okay, we managed to do a study, make a practice change in our institution based on evidence, but now it seemed we could not share this good news with others. We thought we should give up. No one likes rejection, and those rejection letters felt so personal and hurtful. So, after a rejection came, we found it was important to share our feelings, support each other, and gear ourselves up once again.

With that in mind, our team decided to submit our article to one more journal. I guess the adage that the third time is a charm is correct. To all our delight, our manuscript was accepted and published. So our advice to others is to never give up. Keep submitting; you might have the perfect article one journal is looking for. EBP is not as easy as 1-2-3, but stay the course, it will make a difference.

NOTE: Warmest thanks to the APNs that made this journey possible, to the nursing endowment fund for supporting this research study, and to our administration who endorsed our results with the wearing of the nurse badges.

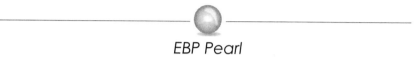

EBP Pearl

Although research and EBP are not easy, find a mentor and keep persisting in your efforts to advance evidence-based care; mentorship and persistence will pay off and make a positive difference in your patients' outcomes.

Suzanne and the Very Big Research Project

–Suzanne Etheredge Alford, ADN, RNC
Lead Staff Nurse NICU, ECMO Specialist and Primer
Children's Health System of Birmingham, Birmingham, Alabama

Some people were born to do research. I was dragged into it kicking and screaming. I have been a neonatal intensive care nurse for over 20 years. It's hard to change. One day our extracorporeal membrane oxygenation (ECMO) coordinator said, "We're a Magnet hospital now. Everyone does evidence-based practice (EBP). We need to do it. Who's with me?" Dead silence. She lost me at EBP. So, very reluctantly and with lots of hand holding, we picked a project, read some articles, reviewed some charts, divided jobs, wrote, charted, graphed, and made a poster. I had poster duty. When we met again at the end, I was asked, "Well, what did you find out?" Without hesitation I answered, "We don't chart enough information." Can you believe it? Nurses don't chart enough data. I actually enjoyed the chart reviews and reading about patients I remembered from several years ago. Some I didn't remember, but my name was all over their chart.

What else did I learn? You can't ask just ONE question. When you search for the answer to your one "burning question," you find yourself asking 10 more questions. What is THE ONE most important thing you need for a successful research project? A mentor. Someone who knows everything that needs to be done, someone who is organized, who can delegate and teach. I had that person. Now, when EBP projects are mentioned, I raise my hand. I love being a part of the process of change. Can you believe I said that?

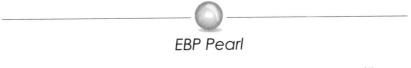

EBP Pearl

EBP mentors get nurses excited about best practice, so either get an EBP mentor or be an EBP mentor.

Creating an Evidence-Based Algorithm for the Prevention and Treatment of Diaper Dermatitis

–Victoria Beall, BSN, RN, CWOCN
Diamond Children's Medical Center at University Medical Center
Tucson, Arizona

I have been a pediatric nurse for more than two decades and have seen my share of diaper dermatitis. Throughout the years, I also have seen many different therapies for the treatment of diaper dermatitis, such as bare bottoms aimed at heat lamps, oxygen being delivered through an adult oxygen mask to the bottom of a baby positioned on his/her belly, cloth diapers, Maalox, or a mixture of Karaya powder and diaper creams smeared on bottoms. I was never sure of the best treatment or the effectiveness of all of these various treatments.

Several years ago, I became a board certified wound, ostomy, and continence nurse (WOCN). Evidence-based practice (EBP) and the use of algorithms were presented hand in hand. One of my goals as a new WOCN for the pediatric units was to develop an evidence-based algorithm for the nurses to prevent and treat diaper dermatitis as a means of standardizing care and to procure appropriate products to be used by the neonatal/pediatric population. Being a new WOCN who was not well known on all the pediatric units, I decided that instead of developing this algorithm myself, I would enlist nurses from each of the pediatric units to form a diaper dermatitis task force to work on this project as a means of "buy-in."

Two multidisciplinary task forces were formed: one in the neonatal intensive care unit (NICU) to address the unique skin issues of the premature infant and one that included a nurse from each of the other pediatric units to address the unique issues of the immunocompromised child, a child with short bowel syndrome, and the older child with incontinence-associated dermatitis (IAD).

The NICU multidisciplinary task force consisted of a NICU night shift staff nurse, a neonatal clinical pharmacist, a nurse discharge coordinator, and a neonatal nurse practitioner. The pediatric task force consisted of staff nurses from the infant toddler unit, the school-age adolescent unit, and the pediatric intensive care unit; pediatric nurse practitioners; a pediatric clinical pharmacist; and patient care technician. My role was to facilitate each task force and to insure that we found and used the best evidence in the algorithm.

The plan was to have nurses each read an article from an evidence-based resource and write an abstract summarizing the findings. Then we as a group would review the abstracts, rate the evidence, and organize the information that we obtained. This was accomplished as intended. However, we encountered the challenge that some of the members of the task force were not familiar with evidence-based practice (EBP) and did not know how to identify evidence-based resources. As a result, only two abstracts were submitted. We brought in a speaker, who was the director of research, to assist us with the process.

Many of the nurses had routines for treating diaper dermatitis that were unit "traditions," and these traditional practices were very dear to them. Some of the nurses resisted looking at the evidence, wanting to put their favorite practices into the algorithm. But we set standards. Everything in the algorithm had to have a rationale, and it needed to be evidence-based. Several nurses from the task force volunteered to find research-based articles and distribute them to the task force. One of the resources that I offered was a book entitled *Neonatal Skin Care*, which is an evidence-based clinical practice guideline in its second edition put out by the Association of Women's Health, Obstetric and Neonatal Nurses (AWHONN). In the book was a chapter on diaper dermatitis. Every clinical practice recommendation listed had a referenced rationale and quality of evidence rating. The nurses in the task force were willing to use this book as a start in creating the evidence-based algorithm. We then looked at other research-based resources that substantiated what we found in the AWHONN guidelines. In using this book, we found that topical ointments were recommended by ingredients and not by brand name, so we needed to find products with the ingredients that were recommended and needed to do away with products that listed ingredients that were recommended to avoid. This became the second part of the process.

To start the second part of the process, we looked at the products that we were currently using in the hospital to see if they met the guidelines that we chose to follow. Then we looked at other products that were on the market. We obtained approval from the director of pediatrics to purchase one of the topical ointments that we understood to fit the guideline.

The next step in the plan was to instruct the staff on how to use the evidence-based algorithm and how to use the products appropriately. We had several inservices and handed out the algorithms to the staff at their gatherings and partnership council meetings. Algorithms were placed in the patient's bedside chart so that the nurses would have easy access to them. The best instruction turned out to be one-on-one instruction with the staff nurse and the WOCN at the bedside of the patient who had diaper dermatitis.

The challenge to date with this process has been with the physicians and licensed independent practitioners who are still ordering products that have ingredients that many of the evidence-based guidelines recommend avoiding. Throughout this process, I felt resistance from some task force members and acknowledged the frustration from several task force members about the time that the process was taking and the loss of some of their favorite "traditions." Although the 7-month process to implement the evidence-based guideline might seem like a long time, the length of time was important for the staff to be exposed to the process and to accept it. The time involved with the process was well worth it.

The Neonatal and Pediatric Algorithms for the Prevention and Treatment for Diaper Dermatitis have been in our unit-based protocols for a year now. As a WOCN nurse, I am consulted on all cases of diaper dermatitis and am finding less severe cases of diaper dermatitis because nurses are now following the evidence-based algorithm for prevention, early intervention, and treatment. This algorithm has empowered nurses to have an evidence-based practice.

EBP Pearl

EBP does not happen overnight—it takes a strong leader and involvement of front-line clinicians in the EBP process to facilitate its success.

Caring and Communication in Nursing: The Experiences of a Nursing Instructor and Seven Nursing Students During a Mental Health Clinical Rotation

–Ileen Craven, MSN, RN
Nursing Instructor, Roxborough Memorial Hospital School of Nursing
Lansdale, Pennsylvania

During the last semester of my nursing school's curriculum, freshman students are educated on caring for mentally ill patients in the classroom and clinical settings. Though therapeutic communication is taught earlier in the curriculum, the school assumes that these techniques will be further developed and that the concepts of caring will be refined during encounters with these patients.

One of the psychiatric clinical facilities assigned is a state hospital for the mentally ill, which is located just outside of a large metropolitan area in the northeast region of the United States. This facility was opened in the late 1800s and in subsequent years has housed thousands of mentally ill patients. Many buildings are now vacant, and its current census is below three hundred, with only four buildings left open to care for general, geriatric, and forensic psychiatric patients.

The patients at this hospital suffer from chronic mental illness and often live there for many years. The majority of nursing students are assigned to clinical facilities that care for the acutely mentally ill patient. Hospital stay in the acute facility is often less than a week. In 2005, when patients were admitted for a diagnosis of depression, the United States government reported an average length of stay as 6.6 days.

Throughout the assigned mental health semester, students participate in clinical for 2 days a week, with the rotation 5 weeks in length. During the first day of orientation, they gain knowledge of the facility from a staff educator. This is followed by the instructor educating them on the requirements of clinical paperwork and on expectations of how to care for the psychiatric patient and asking students about their feelings related to being assigned clinical at a state hospital for the mentally ill. The seven students all expressed feeling deeply frightened, not knowing what to expect, and not sure how to speak to these patients. They couldn't wait until the rotation and school year was over. The median age of these students was early to mid-20s, all expressing a deep interest in nursing since early childhood, but all stipulating that none of them wanted to be psychiatric nurses. Thus began day one of a 5-week journey between a nursing instructor and seven students.

Nursing education is multilayered and filled with many principles and concepts necessary for the success of educating a student on becoming a safe and competent evidence-based practitioner. The more concrete components of nursing education include clinical skills, disease processes, medication administration, and various tasks required to ensure safe patient care. One of the most abstract components for nursing students is the concept of caring. Kapborg and Bertero describe the concept of caring as a process, an interaction that concerns quality, relating to a patient's physical, emotional, and intellectual needs and central to nursing.

A nursing instructor is responsible for educating students that a patient is not defined as a disease, but as a holistic human being with various components that make up the entire person. McGorman and Sultan report that when practitioners care for the mentally ill, they need to incorporate a framework that takes into consideration the mind, body, and entire environment. In caring for the mentally ill, this consideration is paramount because often patients have low self-esteem, feel stigmatized because of diagnoses, and frequently have difficulty in self-expression. According to Rhem, the stigma of mental illness "is the biggest obstacle mental health experts face in helping patients, reducing suicide rates."

The role of the nursing instructor who educates about mental illness includes promoting collaboration between the student and instructor, demonstrating holistic care, and encouraging the student to incorporate critical thinking into patient encounters. To ensure a successful mental health curriculum, the nursing instructor does not have sole responsibility. During the mental health clinical, the ultimate accountability is for the student to be an active and autonomous learner.

An instructor can ease the fear of students caring for the mentally ill patient by using positive attitudes and strategies that incorporate, among other factors, the clinical picture. The clinical picture of patients at the state hospital is diverse. Patients who reside on the assigned clinical unit range in age from late 20s to early 70s, with some having lived there as little as 6 months to as long as 40 years. Most are diagnosed with DSM IV-TR criteria necessary for schizophrenia. Some have no family support, whereas others remain close to members of their families. There are more males than females, and many reside quietly amongst one another, with little incidents of violence despite the diagnosis of schizophrenia. Patients on the unit still may exhibit the ever-persistent auditory and/or visual hallucinations, fixed delusions, and feelings of social isolation thatoften are related to the positive and negative symptoms of the disease. Yet, despite being diagnosed with schizophrenia, these patients display moments of joy, laughter, and happiness.

In the effort to further humanize these patients, during preconference on the second assigned day of clinical, the instructor began to tell life stories of various patients who reside at this facility. The instructor had no script, used no chart, and had no agenda. In communicating to these students that these patients were human beings, the instructor attempted to put a face on a disease and holistic components on a patient, rather than focus on the signs and symptoms causing hospitalization. Narratives often assist in bringing down barriers and stigmas, assisting in communication, and changing the role of perceptions and ideas about illness. With this in mind, the students heard of four patients residing at this state hospital. Here is one patient's story:

C. is a woman in her late 40s. During most of her childhood she was the victim of sexual abuse caused by both parents and several of her 17 siblings. Her mother sold her into prostitution and once placed a hot curling iron in her vagina to punish her. During adolescence, she began experiencing auditory hallucinations, the voice of a male who commanded her to (1) tear both of her eyes out, which she did and which caused her blindness; (2) push a passenger in front of a train, which she did and that person died; and (3) murder her own child, whose father was her brother. For years she had lived in and out of mental hospitals except for the last 4 years, where this state facility was her home.

Despite a lifelong history of violence, she has performed no violent acts since residing there. She is employed through the hospital's vocational services and has had decreases in hallucinations and exhibits laughter and happiness at various times. She also has made friends among certain other patients, particularly J., whom she calls "Mom."

Though C.'s story may have been the most horrific and sad, the remaining stories also were about patients who found that the disease of schizophrenia affected their abilities to lead "normal" lives in society and influenced their abilities to function socially, occupationally, and economically. The patients who resided on this unit were not like the students who would become nurses, get married, have children, and live productive lives in society. Yet they remained human beings who still expressed wishes to somehow fit into societal demands and function within the norms of life.

The four stories told by a nursing instructor with seven students present in the room were followed by tears, questions, and a sense of these students' fears alleviated. The students then expressed their willingness to be a part of the experience in caring for and getting to know these patients. They now wanted to become a positive and vital element of these patients' lives, even if for only 5 weeks. No longer did they see these patients as an assigned diagnosis, but rather as whole human beings whose lives were shattered by schizophrenia.

These nursing students spent a great deal of the clinical day talking to patients, listening to their preferences and values, and adopting ones that would be their primary patient during those 5 weeks. Though the students were asked to complete clinical paperwork, which included mental status examinations, process recordings, psychiatric nursing assessments, and care plans, the students did not approach the patients as clinicians just looking to get their paperwork done. During the 5 weeks the students talked to patients as if they were speaking to anyone else they would meet.

Aside from talking to patients, students and the instructor attended treatment team meetings, which showed collaboration and communication among disciplinary teams. The team was composed of individualized patients, nurses, physicians, social workers, recreation therapists, and psychologists. Interdisciplinary teams have a great importance in health care by showing the diversity of each discipline, the perspectives brought in by each team member, and the ability to look at a patient's physical and psychosocial needs through effective communication and open dialogue. This was the first time students saw and participated in treatment team meetings. They expressed an understanding of their importance and necessity in providing a continuum of care for the patient diagnosed with a mental and/or physical illness. Aside from group activities and meetings the students played games with patients, attended workshops with patients who were able to work, sang and danced with patients who loved these activities, and learned to advocate for patients who they felt might have been unfairly treated or not listened to by staff members.

The last day of clinical was set aside as a time to throw the patients a party and say goodbye. The instructor and students supplied the patients with soft pretzels, water, ice, music, and dancing. More importantly feelings were shared on how valuable this experience clinical was and how sad everyone was to leave. Most impressive were C.'s tears when she realized she would never again see Teresa, the student who spent 5 weeks getting to know her and becoming a part of her life.

During 5 weeks, the journey of one nursing instructor and seven nursing students began at a state psychiatric facility. Despite the original fears and apprehensions exhibited and reported by these students, the lessons they learned were invaluable. The patients diagnosed with mental illness were seen as beyond a set of clinical criteria and as human beings with many parts that make up the whole person. The students also learned to integrate patients' preferences and values into their evidence-based decision-making, enhance their therapeutic communication skills, listen and remain silent when necessary, advocate for patients who may have no clear methods of communication, work within an interdisciplinary team, and practice caring with pureness of heart.

EBP Pearl

All patients deserve to have their preferences and values integrated into evidence-based care.

Helping Veterans Find Hope

–Frederick H. Osborne, MS, PMHNP
Veterans Affairs Medical Center
Canandaigua, New York

"You know, this program saved my life. I'd probably be dead right now if I didn't come here." This comment came from a combat veteran who had already survived a war. The statement made me smile, but did not surprise me. I had grown accustomed to similar comments from veterans who had participated in our Partial Hospital Program (PHP). The PHP is a short duration, intensive group therapy program for veterans with a mental illness. The intent of the program is to help veterans in the VA system manage their symptoms and learn new skills. Anecdotally, we had been hearing many stories from veterans in our program at the Canandaigua VA in Upstate New York about their remarkable recovery from mental illness. Our program had evolved over several years under the guidance of our nurse manager. The groups and classes were developed utilizing evidence-based practices in mental health treatment. Staff members were encouraged to seek out educational experiences in specific evidence-based practices and incorporate what they had learned into groups. Our all-RN staff had received many comments from veterans about the usefulness of the program, as well as biweekly written evaluations from veterans that were generally glowing. But the question was, "How do we document and verify what we knew to be effective?"

I recalled learning in graduate school that all nursing staff were encouraged to participate in evidence-based practice and that the process was strengthened when they participated in measuring outcomes and documenting them in whatever clinical area they worked. Our PHP staff decided to start a database of our program participants and began entering data on an Excel spreadsheet that resided on a shared disk drive. Any member of our staff could enter data, and we did so a little at a time. We listed every participant and decided on demographic data that would be useful to track for further refining of the program. Our staff chose several outcomes measures that we thought would be helpful for outcomes management.

The mission of the program, in part, was to prevent admissions to inpatient psychiatric units. A dramatic example of the power of the program to affect change in this area came when a former participant returned for a visit. "I had a psychotic break," he said, "but for the first time in 30 years, I didn't need to go into the hospital. I learned that I had choices, and I managed the situation on my own." So, one outcomes measure became the admissions to inpatient psychiatric units within 60 days of discharge for those who had completed our program. Additionally, we had been using an informal mood-rating scale at the beginning of the program day and at the end of the day. This gave the staff and veteran an indication of progress throughout the day. Over time, it also gave an indication of progress over the course of the program. This information was readily available, so we decided to use this mood rating from the beginning of the program to the end as another outcomes measure. Although this was not a standardized measure, it did give an idea of the veteran's subjective perception of mood. We then thought that we might strengthen this measure by correlating it to a standardized measure of mood. We added the Quick Inventory of Depressive Symptoms, or QIDS, as an outcomes measure. This self-report measure was done at admission and at discharge.

Our database grew slowly over time. It wasn't hard or time-consuming, just a few minutes a day. Every staff member could contribute, which meant that every staff member was a part of the outcomes project. When we had collected a year's data, we transferred the information to a statistics program and ran some tests. The demographic data was somewhat surprising. Although we worked with small groups each day, it was interesting to see "the big picture" and how the population as a whole looked. Furthermore, the demographic information could be used to guide the programming that we were using.

Our outcomes measures were not a surprise. They showed that the veterans who were treated in our program made statistically significant improvements in our outcomes measures. Pleased with the results, we asked ourselves what we could do with this information. We wanted a venue to present this information. Our facility nurse executive suggested a poster presentation at a national conference that was fast approaching. An abstract was submitted and accepted. A poster was developed, printed on an 8-by-4-foot piece of vinyl, and escorted to Indianapolis, IN, for presentation. Physicians and nurses from VAs across the country could see the work and success of a small group of nurses from our facility in treating those with a mental illness.

The effect of this on the PHP staff has been subtle, but significant. I have noticed an increase in staff camaraderie. Each staff member seems to have an increased respect for the work of others, and staff members have more appreciation for the strengths of other staff members when discussing specific treatment issues. We discuss treatment aspects for veterans more as a team instead of as individual providers. The veterans benefit, and the staff enjoy their work.

Last week I sat with another staff member in a quiet area and listened as a veteran tearfully exclaimed that he was finally able to grieve for a loss that had occurred 17 years ago. He credited the staff and program for giving him the skills to accomplish this task. "I kept it all inside because I didn't know how to do it any different," he said.

Another veteran strolled by and entered into the conversation. "I know what you mean," he said. "I've learned stuff here that I've been using to handle my anger. I've never been able to do that before." He too had experienced a relief of symptoms and felt confident that he could use the skills he had learned in the PHP to help himself in the future. It was one of those moments in nursing when you know that you are a part of something that is making a difference in people's lives. The exciting part, though, is that we have documented the effectiveness of our program and presented it for others to see. The PHP is based on evidenced-based practices, and now we have the data to demonstrate that what we are accomplishing with this specific population is clearly shown in the outcomes data. We are adding to the body of knowledge for evidence-based practices in the treatment of veterans with mental illnesses.

EBP Pearl

Evaluation and dissemination are critical steps of the EBP process; don't forget them!

The Introduction of an Evidence-Based Change: Sensory Modulation in Behavioral Health

–Joan S. Parker-Dias, MSN, RN-BC, APRN
Clinical Nurse Specialist for Behavioral Health
Queen's Medical Center, Honolulu, Hawaii

Mental health programs have been using seclusion and restraints for years to manage out-of-control behavior. Many organizations have been concerned about the negative effects of these interventions. The Substance Abuse and Mental Health Services Administration and the Center for Mental Health Services have developed best practice approaches to prevent seclusion and restraints in mental health.

The focus of this story is the difficulty of obtaining organizational change and the buy-in of the staff involved with the change. As I tell the story, I will briefly outline the national initiative for eliminating seclusion and restraints, define sensory modulation, and discuss challenges experienced in initiating sensory modulation. Some of those challenges are (a) experiences with initiating change; (b) being a change agent; (c) encountering resistance towards change; and (d) maintaining motivation of the change and motivation for future changes.

The Child and Adolescent Mental Health Division in Hawaii successfully obtained a grant to be part of the initiative that is focused on eliminating seclusion and restraints. The child/adolescent psychiatric unit in Honolulu, where I work, was fortunate to benefit from this grant. This process required a monumental organizational shift that began with training our staff in the six core strategies that focus on trauma-informed/coercion-free care. I was one of the lead facilitators who brought some of the practices to our unit. The six core strategies involve change at all levels of the organization, requiring everyone's support for the initiative to be successful. The six core strategies are (1) leadership towards organizational change; (2) use of data to inform practice; (3) workforce development; (4) use of prevention tools; (5) supporting consumer advocate roles; and (6) debriefing tools.

As part of this initiative, our unit began to use sensory modulation, which has been shown to be an effective alternative to the use of seclusion and restraints. Sensory modulation is a person's ability to respond to a sensory stimulation in a positive manner. Tina, an occupational therapist, designed a quality improvement study to examine the possible benefits of the use of sensory modulation with children, adolescents, and adults in an inpatient psychiatric unit. With the positive outcomes of her project, the organization added sensory modulation techniques into their programs. These changes resulted in increased client satisfaction, decreased use of medication, and decreased rates of seclusion and restraints post-initiation.

My experience with sensory modulation involved initiating it into two programs, an inpatient child/adolescent unit and an acute adult unit. A change agent is a person who leads change by defining, researching, planning, building support, and selecting volunteers to be part of the team. In the child/adolescent unit, I was the lead facilitator (change agent) in developing sensory modulation rooms. After we established a committee on the child/adolescent unit to initiate sensory modulation, occupational staff from the adult unit wanted to join our committee so they could initiate sensory modulation on their unit. For a successful project, staff must be informed about the initiative, a core group of staff must be involved in the planning, and the initiative must be supported by all levels of management. The staff of the child/adolescent unit had been educated regarding the national initiative and had been exposed to the six core strategies. In contrast, the adult unit staff and leadership only heard informally about the initiative and were not formally trained regarding the core strategies.

The effects of poor communication were evident almost immediately as the adult unit staff were reluctant to get involved with the sensory modulation committee and lacked motivation to use sensory techniques. Many of the child/adolescent staff volunteered to be on the committee and many were asking for more items and techniques to try with clients to help with de-escalation.

One article on initiating change discussed the importance of placing the change agent within the system. I was placed at the service-delivery level, but the macrosystem was not set up on the adult unit and the leadership of the adult unit did not support this initiative at first. The staff were not informed nor prepared for this change, which affected the launch of this project. During the Behavioral Health Division meeting, which included members from the leadership of the child/adolescent and adult psychiatric units, the initiative was discussed and the importance of involvement at all levels of the organization was reinforced. At this point, the development of the sensory rooms was postponed until mass education of all adult psychiatric staff was completed. This postponement also occurred because the hospital had another competing initiative, which was the transition into a new hospital-wide computer system. The staff was already overwhelmed with the new integrative computer system. It was decided to educate adult unit staff on sensory modulation over a 3-month period to avoid overburdening and overwhelming them.

A leadership team was charged with leading the sensory modulation change, getting affected staff involved, and most importantly communicating the plan for initiating the change. The lack of communication on the adult psychiatric units about the planned change negatively impacted the use of the sensory modulation techniques and the development of the sensory rooms. The lack of managerial support for prioritizing these efforts and identifying mechanisms to back the initiative was another factor that might have contributed to staffs' reluctance to get involved in the process. Furthermore, many adult staff verbalized fear for their safety regarding the change from focusing on negative behavior to focusing on providing positive reinforcement, as in sensory modulation. Past practice would isolate an agitated patient in the seclusion room where they had nothing but a mattress on the floor, as opposed to the various items that would be found in a sensory room. Staff felt it was unsafe to put an escalated patient into a sensory room.

It took a lot of education, communication, and positive examples of successful cases to slowly move the staff towards using sensory modulation. Three of the staff who were very negative about this initiative had positive responses after they tried sensory modulation techniques. These staff members then became strong advocates for its use. Currently, staff on the adult unit continue to be leery to use sensory modulation, and we continue to work with this group. On the child/adolescent unit, seclusion and restraint events decreased from an average of 20 events per month down to 2 to 3 events per month. For 3 months none of the child/adolescent programs had any events. The next step will be to develop the use of sensory modulation within different programs, by setting a clear vision and plan that is communicated to a strong team who is charged with making the change.

NOTE: Special thanks to contributors: Joan S. Parker-Dias, MSN, RN-BC, APRN; Chuck St. Louis, MSN, RN, APRN; Carol Hanakahi, RN; Lyndell Shunk, RN-BC; Justin Mullen, OTR; Lisa Minchew, CRT; and Kathryn Shawhan, OTR.

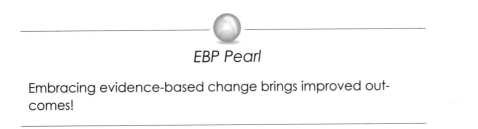

EBP Pearl

Embracing evidence-based change brings improved outcomes!

At Last

–Julia Peden Wetmore, PhD, RN, CNE
Assistant Professor
Western Carolina University, Cullowhee, North Carolina

I have a hate-love relationship with nursing research. I was a nursing student 30 years ago, way back in the dark ages, back before the Internet, back before computers. Back then, we had to trot over to a university library; sit down with CINAHL or the Index Medicus (precursor to Medline, which used to be on shelves in actual volumes); look up citations of articles; write down the citations; go find the articles in the stacks of periodicals; and then copy them, paying for the articles at 10 cents a sheet. We read the articles, decided (based on the little we knew about research, the patient, and the disease process) if we could use the article. We then incorporated the suggested interventions into our carefully crafted nursing care plan. I often used recommendations from studies that I knew could not really be generalized to my patient and that I suspected, based on my limited knowledge of nursing research, were not very well done.

I understood so little about research and knew so little about patient care that trying to fit the intervention to my care plan was mostly a shot in the dark. I knew that there was no easy way to find an appropriate and safe plan for my patient from the vast ocean of literature before me, and that I had no way to be reasonably sure I had found the best option. If I couldn't do it, I suspected that nobody else could either.

After graduation, I left the world of academia for a few years and concentrated on my clinical skills. I worked at a children's hospital on a critical care unit. I worked really hard, long days and even harder, longer nights. I became a good pediatric critical care nurse during those years, but I don't think I looked up a single research study or entered a single library. I occasionally looked up something in a textbook and depended on my peers, my supervisors, and physicians for information.

Then, I was on to graduate school where I learned to do a complete literature review—very tedious. I made my first and last C in my MSN program, in the research and statistics course, which I despised. I studied research and/or statistics only when it was required, and I made sure that it was very seldom.

So, in my doctoral program, I needed to go back and learn the research and statistics I failed to learn at the master's level. I found a wonderful statistics teacher who helped me catch up and taught me to love statistics (a miracle). He got me over my math anxiety, and I learned to understand the research process. I saw the beauty and symmetry of a well-done study. I learned to apply research to patient care situations in the form of evidence-based care. Most of my doctoral work, however, was done in the library. I had a personal computer for word and data processing, but there was still no such thing as the Internet.

My first job after earning my PhD was teaching research to RN to BSN students. I loved it. I taught my students to be unafraid of research. They wrote papers and proposed studies, making connections between research and practice. I enjoyed teaching them to think about problems in patient care and how they might solve the problems by designing studies to answer research questions.

It was 1993, and I had two small sons. I was newly separated from my husband, and I found that I needed to stay home to be with my children. I left nursing education and did not return to work until 2004. During that time, a remarkable thing happened—the Internet.

When my sons were small, I did not know much about the Internet. We got a computer after my boys entered elementary school, and I thought I kept a pretty close watch over it. Even though the computer was in the middle of our family room, one summer afternoon my oldest son put "naked people" in as a search term. Out came naked people—lots of them. I got a "net nanny" after that.

The nursing research world changed dramatically with the advent of the Internet. Basing practice on research was finally possible. Given the right circumstances, a nurse could actually find the very best practice recommendations for a specific patient and insert them into a plan of care. Remarkable, but still developing.

EBP is now much more refined, but some problems are still with us in 2011. Nurses continue to need to know how to find and extract best practices from the literature, and they need to know how to change current clinical practices. But they are learning! I am able to teach my RN to BSN students to base practice on evidence, and this excites me, a 50-something nursing professor who was once a frustrated senior nursing student.

Each semester, my students finish the semester with a real-life "EBP project." Students identify a nursing problem in their practice and find evidence to solve the problem. Here are some wonderful examples of the initial questions and the outcomes of our EBP projects that were completed in 2010:

> *"In patients with congestive heart failure (CHF), how does telehealth monitoring effectively reduce hospital readmissions?" This home health nurse was able to demonstrate that home monitoring effectively reduces hospital readmissions for congestive heart failure.*

> *"In mild to moderately dehydrated pediatric patients less than 5 years of age, how effective is oral rehydration when compared to the administration of intravenous fluids, in the treatment of acute, viral gastroenteritis?" This pediatric ED nurse was committed to demonstrating that oral rehydration is as effective as intravenous, and she found the appropriate evidence.*

> *"In hospitalized patients diagnosed with sleep apnea, is supplemental oxygen an effective alternative to CPAP?" This student was concerned that patients admitted to her unit without their at-home CPAP units were at increased risk for heart attack and stroke, a fact supported in the literature. She found evidence for providing CPAP machines for this inpatient population.*

"What is the best way to maintain good oral health in developmentally disabled adults?" This student designed a program for oral care in a tertiary care facility.

"In school-age children, do nit-free policies decrease the spread of head lice?" This school nurse was concerned that children were missing too many days of school because of lice. She helped to change her school system's head lice policy.

"In post-mastectomy patients, will timely information about upper extremity rehabilitation decrease impairments, not only by providing education on strategies for preventing impairment but also by contributing to the knowledge base underlying the strategies?" This breast cancer navigator went on to design a new teaching program for breast cancer patients based on her project.

Every semester now, I get to introduce another group of nurses to evidence-based nursing practice. I look forward to discussing their ideas and leading them to the right question for the patient care situation. I insist that they begin with patient care rather than nursing administration or education, because that's where they learn the process the best, at the bedside. And after all, that's where we all begin learning to be nurses, at the bedside.

I'm so glad I finally fell in love with nursing research, and I'm so glad I have an opportunity to help other nurses learn to love it. I think that EBP makes nursing research so much easier to love.

At last.

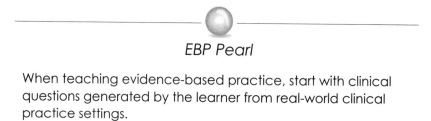

EBP Pearl

When teaching evidence-based practice, start with clinical questions generated by the learner from real-world clinical practice settings.

Reigniting a Passion for Nursing

–Karen Balakas, PhD, RN, CNE
Goldfarb School of Nursing at Barnes-Jewish College
St. Louis, Missouri

In my role as nursing faculty, I had attended numerous conferences and educational seminars over the past three decades. And, as with most attendees, I usually took away something that was perhaps interesting and that I might want to learn more about or use in my work setting. I was looking forward to a presentation at our local hospital in the fall of 2005 by Drs. Bernadette Melnyk and Ellen Fineout-Overholt on evidence-based practice (EBP). This was a new concept for me, and I wasn't sure it was going to be meaningful to me as an educator. But EBP seemed important for nursing practice, so December 2005 found me in the first cohort to take the EBP Mentorship program at Arizona State University. I expected to learn all about EBP, but I was not at all prepared to be completely changed!

Following an intensive week at ASU, during which time I worked with two colleagues to incorporate EBP as we redesigned our entire RN-to-BSN curriculum, I became a member of another hospital-based team dedicated to teaching EBP. We christened ourselves the "Evidence Equals Excellence" group, and in February 2006, we began conducting three to four EBP workshops annually throughout our hospital system. At this time, we have introduced EBP to hundreds of staff nurses and have seen its impact in the care that is delivered through projects and revised policies. Over the past 4 years, we have continually improved the 2-day workshop, and our teaching team has grown to welcome additional nurses who have completed the EBP Mentorship program. Furthermore, we started an EBP Fellowship within our large, academic hospital for nurses who have taken the initial workshop and want to increase their knowledge and EBP skills.

The nurse educator in me knew that it was imperative that I also change how I taught research courses to both undergraduate and graduate students. It was difficult at first to let go of all my sacred cows! (Really, do we need to know all the ways you can go about getting a sample?) Making research all about using evidence in practice and connecting it to our world as practitioners was exciting, and students responded enthusiastically. The undergraduate students partnered with others in their clinical area or in the community to develop and appraise a PICO question, whereas the graduate students designed an EBP project for implementation in their work setting.

In 2008, I began a joint appointment through the college with two area hospitals, which offered another opportunity to teach and apply EBP. In my new role, I direct nursing research and EBP in both facilities. In the academic hospital, I have revised the beginning EBP curriculum and mentored several nurses in their projects. Now I am establishing a new position within the Professional Practice Department for an advanced practice nurse committed to facilitating and intensely monitoring EBP projects. Hopefully, this nurse will become a reality by the end of the year! Working in a large community hospital has given me the chance to build an EBP and a research department from the beginning. With administrative support, 18 nurses have completed a 10-week EBP program in 2 years. With over half the nurses finishing their projects and presenting locally, regionally, and nationally, my real joy is in seeing their accomplishments. I know what it means for the patients they care for and for their colleagues who are then able to deliver evidence-based care, too.

Becoming a champion for evidence-based practice has made a tremendous difference in my personal and professional life. It has opened doors for me as an educator and as a practicing nurse. Creating workshops, developing curricula, writing articles, and conducting research about EBP have all contributed to reenergizing my academic career. Applying EBP skills to my own nursing practice in caring for ill neonates has reignited my passion for nursing. Years ago when I was completing graduate school, one of my teachers said that "nursing diagnosis" was important to her, and that she was going to dedicate the rest of her career to it. I now know what she meant. I now know what it means to feel such enthusiasm for something and to want to devote my energy to sharing it with others.

Epilogue

Now that you have been inspired by these heartwarming real-life stories of clinicians changing patients' experiences and outcomes in health care, changing systems, and changing "the way we've always done it," follow the advice of Yoda, the famous *Star Wars* Jedi master, who wisely said, "Do or do not . . . there is no try." Dreams without execution will not come to reality, so dream big to launch innovative projects and studies that will make a positive difference in your patients' lives; take risks, keeping in mind that success is going from one failure to the next with enthusiasm; and persist through the character-builders until you achieve those dreams. We believe in you—you can do it!

Bern Melnyk & Ellen Fineout-Overholt

Index

D

E